MCAT Practice
Verbal Reasoning Passages
Volume I

For in-depth MCAT, GRE, and GMAT training and publications visit:

www.ivyhallreview.com

MCAT Practice
Verbal Reasoning Passages

Volume I

Compiled by
Charles A. Chaney

Edited by
Charles L. Chaney

IVYHALL REVIEW

MCAT ® is a registered trademark of the American Association of Medical Colleges

Published by IvyHall Review,
31130 Rancho Viejo Road
San Juan Capistrano, CA 92675

ISBN 13 978-0-9816721-1-3
ISBN 10 0-9816721-1-6

Printed in the United States of America.

10 9 8 7 6 5 4 3 2 1

Table of Contents

About This Book

As an aspiring healthcare professional, you are well aware of the extensive preparation needed to achieve a high score on the MCAT, especially on Verbal Reasoning. Unfortunately, many students perform poorly on this section every year. Students who score very high on Verbal Reasoning invest great time and energy in order to be prepared. Studies show that students who practice with challenging and difficult reading material are usually the most successful.

We believe that the harder your practice tests, the better your chances of securing an impressive MCAT score.

With this in mind, the 50 passages presented here span the same topics as those of the real MCAT at the same level of difficulty.

These 50 Passages are divided into seven complete 1-hour Verbal Reasoning exams, each containing seven passages. In addition, we have included a Warm-up Passage to get you started.

The latter portion of the book is dedicated to Answers and Explanations. Please take the time to understand your mistakes, as well as your correct answers.

Good reading!

About the Author

Charles A. Chaney has taught many clients how to maximize reading comprehension and memory, having pioneered a new approach to reading called Neuro-Visual Programming. After earning his master's degree from Johns Hopkins University, he began teaching students and professionals to prepare for a number of entrance exams.

His advice is simple. Dedicate the time and effort today, face the most difficult challenges, and your mind will excel without limit tomorrow.

Practice, practice, practice. Success will follow.

Charles can be reached at *verbalbook@gmail.com.*

MCAT Tips:
Timing and Pacing

The table below summarizes the various parts of the MCAT with information about timing and the number of questions per section.

Test Section	Time	Details
Non-Disclosure Agreement	10 min	required
Tutorial	10 min	optional
Physical Sciences	70 min	52 questions
Break	10 min	optional
Verbal Reasoning	60 min	40 questions
Break	10 min	optional
Writing Sample	60 min	2 essays
Break	10 min	optional
Biological Sciences	70 min	52 questions
Void Question	5 min	required
Survey	10 min	optional

Total time = 5 hours, 25 min

PACING ON VERBAL REASONING

You have 60 minutes on the VR section

There are 7 PASSAGES with 40 QUESTIONS

This equates to 8.5 MINUTES per passage

(each passage contain 5 to 7 Questions)

That means you should aim to read a passage in 3.5 minutes,

leaving 5 minutes to answer questions.

SUGGESTED PACING as the clock counts down from 60:00 is as follows:

MINUTE 60:00   BEGIN PASSAGE I

MINUTE 51:00   BEGIN PASSAGE II

MINUTE 43:00   BEGIN PASSAGE III

MINUTE 34:00   BEGIN PASSAGE IV

MINUTE 26:00   BEGIN PASSAGE V

MINUTE 17:00   BEGIN PASSAGE VI

MINUTE 09:00   BEGIN PASSAGE VII

VERBAL REASONING

Verbal Reasoning, arguably the most difficult section of the MCAT and the one feared most, evaluates the ability to comprehend and apply information presented in passages that are typically 600 words in length. The passages are taken from scholarly articles found in the **humanities, social sciences**, and various areas of the **natural sciences**.

Following each passage are five to seven questions of varying difficulty. Some questions assess your fundamental comprehension of the text, while others require you to analyze information, evaluate the validity of an argument, determine the opinion of an author, identify implied ideas, or apply knowledge to other contexts. This section also tests your ability to read passages and answer questions in a rapid manner under pressure.

The list below provides a quick overview of the kinds of passages frequently encountered. Many libraries organize their book collections around these categories, or ones very similar to them.

- Anthropology
- Economic Theory
- Humanities
- Literary Theory
- Natural Science
- Philosophy of Science
- Political Science
- Psychology
- Art Criticism
- Sociology

THE COMPUTER

You will see that your screen is divided into two vertical halves. On the left half will appear the passage. You will be able to scroll up and down to read it in its entirety. On the right half will appear the questions. You will also be able to scroll up and down to see every question, and the two halves can scroll independently of each other.

The computer does allow examinees to advance forward or backward through neighboring passages without having to answer questions. You can also open a master page that lists all questions, and by selecting the corresponding question, you can open the passage containing that specific question.

Verbal Reasoning Warm-up Passage

Time: 8.5 Minutes
Questions 1 - 6

WARM-UP PASSAGE

DIRECTIONS: There are seven passages in the Verbal Reasoning test. Each passage is followed by five to seven questions. Pace yourself and select the one best answer to each question.

Warm-up Passage (Questions 1 - 6)

Among the acts sanctioned by International Law, none is more worthy of a philosopher's or a philanthropist's attention than the "pacific blockade." The credit for the institution belongs to all the great civilized communities, but for its pleasant designation the world is indebted to the eminent jurist M. Hautefeuille—a countryman of the ingenious Dr. Guillotin. It denotes "a blockade exercised by a great Power for the purpose of bringing pressure to bear on a weaker State, without actual war. That it is an act of violence, and therefore in the nature of war, is undeniable"; but, besides its name, it possesses certain features which distinguish it advantageously from ordinary war.

First, instead of the barbarous effusion of blood and swift destruction which open hostilities entail, the pacific blockade achieves its ends by more refined and leisurely means: one is not shocked by the unseemly sights of a battlefield, and the wielder of the weapon has time to watch its effects as they develop: he can see the victim going through the successive stages of misery— debility, languor, exhaustion—until the final point is reached; and as his scientific curiosity is gratified by the gradual manifestation of the various symptoms, so his moral sense is fortified by the struggle between a proud spirit and an empty stomach—than which life can offer no more ennobling spectacle.

Then, unlike crude war, the pacific blockade automatically strikes the nation at which it is aimed on its weakest side first: instead of having to begin with its manhood, one begins with its old men, its women, and its infants. The merits of this form of attack are evident: many a man who would boldly face starvation himself, may be reasonably expected to flinch at the prospect of a starving mother, wife, or child.

Lastly, whilst in war the assailant must inevitably suffer as well as inflict losses, the pacific blockade renders him absolutely exempt from all risk. For "it can only be employed as a measure of coercion by maritime Powers able to bring into action such vastly superior forces to those the resisting State can dispose of, that resistance is out of the question."

In brief, the pacific blockade is not war, but a kind of sport, as safe as coursing, and to the educated mind much more interesting. The interest largely depends on the duration of the blockade, and its duration on the victims' physical and moral resources…

Next to bread, the most prominent article of Greek diet is fish. The French, who in their treatment of this neutral nation gave evidence of a thoroughness and efficiency such as they did not always display in their operations against the enemy, saw to it that this source of subsistence also should, within the measure of their ability, fail their victims. French cruisers stopped the fishing-smacks and asked if their community had joined the Rebellion. When the answer was in the negative, they sank the vessel and confiscated the tackle, often accompanying the robbery of property with violence on the persons of the owners and abuse of their sovereign. To the wretched fishermen's protests, the French commanders replied: "If you want to be left alone, you have only to drive out your King."

1. The author's central thesis is that:

A. in wartime, an alternative to fighting battles exists.
B. the pacific blockade is a kind of sport.
C. coercion by maritime force is superior to open hostilities.
D. blockades can be more effective than swift destruction.

2. The use of the pacific blockade would have what expected effect on a nation?

    I.   Dramatic increase in unemployment.
    II.   Extensive growth of the indigent population.
    III.   Starvation of animals.

A. I only
B. III only
C. I and II only
D. I, II and III

3. The author suggests that the ultimate object of the blockade is to:

A. cause widespread starvation.
B. propagate rebellion.
C. deplete physical and moral resources.
D. acquire control of a nation.

4. According to the passage, a nation can enact a blockade once it:

A. becomes a maritime power.
B. declares war on another nation.
C. surpasses the resisting nation in force.
D. achieves a favorable economy.

5. A blockade would first cause the cessation of all maritime traffic, followed by what effect on the recipient nation?

A. Cessation of industry, followed by rising poverty.
B. Rise in poverty, followed by cessation of industry.
C. Rise in disease, followed by cessation of industry.
D. Rise in starvation, followed by a cessation of industry.

6. Which of the following statements, if true, would most *weaken* the author's claim that blockade is not war, but a kind of sport?

A. Blockades affect the strongest side of the opposing nation first.
B. The assailant inevitably suffers losses.
C. Maritime fleets enforcing the blockade engage in hostilities with the opposing nation.
D. Blockades cause swift destruction of opposing nations that are weak.

———————————————————

STOP.

Verbal Reasoning Test 1

Time: 60 Minutes
Questions 1 - 40

VERBAL REASONING

DIRECTIONS: There are seven passages in the Verbal Reasoning test. Each passage is followed by five to seven questions. Pace yourself and select the one best answer to each question.

Passage I (Questions 1 - 5)

Immense numbers of these storage cists are found in the canyon, some of them with masonry so roughly executed that it is difficult to discriminate between the old pueblo and the modern Navaho work. Sometimes these cists or small rooms form part of a village, more often they are attached to the cliff outlooks, and not infrequently they stand alone on sites overlooking the lands whose product they contained. It is probable that many of the cliff outlooks themselves were used quite as much for temporary storage as for habitations during the farming season. These two uses, although quite distinct, do not conflict with each other. Doubtless many excellent sites, now marked only by the remains of storage cists, were occupied also during the summer as outlooks without the erection of any house structures. Some of the modern pueblos now use temporary shelters of brush for outlooks.

It is not meant that the crops when gathered were placed in these cists and kept there until used. The harvest was, as a rule, permanently stored in the home villages, and the cists were used only for temporary storage. Doubtless the old practice resembled somewhat that followed by the Navaho today. The harvest is gathered at the proper time and what is not eaten at once is hidden away in cists of old or modern construction. If it is well hidden, the grain may remain in the cists for a long time if not withdrawn for consumption; but as a rule it is taken away a few months later.

The storage of water was so seldom attempted, or perhaps so seldom necessary, that only one example of a reservoir was found. If the cliff ruins were defensive structures, a supply of water must have been kept in them, and where this requirement was common, as it would be under the hypothesis, certainly some receptacle other than jars of pottery would be provided. Few, if any, of the cliff outlooks are so situated that a supply of water could be procured without descending to the stream bed, and without a supply of water the most impregnable site in the canyon would have little value.

The number of burial cists in the canyon is remarkable; there are hundreds of them. Practically every ruin whose walls are still standing contains one or more, some have eight or ten. They are all of Navaho origin and in many of them the remains of Navaho dead may still be seen. Possibly the Navaho taboo of their own dead has brought about the partial taboo of the cliff dwellers' remains which prevails, and which is an element that must be taken into account in any discussion of the antiquity of the ruins. As a whole the Navaho burial cists are much more difficult of access than the ruins, and some of them appear to be now really inaccessible, a statement which can be made of but few ruins. Some of them appear to have been reached from above. The agility and dexterity of the Navaho in climbing the cliffs is remarkable, and possibly some of the sites now apparently inaccessible are not so considered by them. As before stated, there are a number of Navaho foot trails out of the canyon, where shallow pits or holes have been pecked in the rock as an aid in the more difficult places, and similar aids were

GO ON TO THE NEXT PAGE.

often employed to afford access to storage and burial cists.

The pits in the rock are so much worn by atmospheric erosion that the ascent now is very dangerous. The cove or ledge to which they lead is about halfway up the cliff, and on it are a number of cists, one of them still intact, with a doorway. The masonry consists of large slabs of sandstone set on edge, sometimes irregularly one above another, the whole being roughly plastered inside and out. About 200 yards farther up the cove, on the same side, there is a series of foot holes leading to a small cave about halfway up, and thence upward and probably out of the canyon. They are probably of Navaho origin.

1. The author's major thesis is that:

A. Native Americans used cists for several key purposes.
B. The Navaho treated the dead in a remarkable manner.
C. The Navaho utilized cists in a number of ways that often overlapped in function.
D. The Navaho built cists for specific purposes.

2. Which of the following assertions is NOT clearly supported by historical evidence provided by the passage author?

A. Water was seldom stored.
B. Some Navaho storage cists could not be differentiated from those of old pueblo.
C. The Navaho respected their dead.
D. Navaho storage cists were also used for habitation.

3. The author treats the idea of the antiquity of the Navaho ruins as:

A. difficult to access.
B. credible and sacred to the culture.
C. inseparable from the taboo of the dead.
D. evidence for the use of cists as sites of temporary storage.

4. Which of the following inferences is justified by information in the passage?

A. The Navaho believed in some form of afterlife.
B. Storage and habitation were a priority for the Navaho.
C. A similar people, the old pueblo, came before the Navaho.
D. Some catastrophic event struck the Navaho people.

5. The author of the passage seems to hold the opinion that:

A. The Navaho possessed large containers for water storage.
B. Members of the Navaho were tall and fit.
C. The Navaho were attacked often by invaders.
D. Many civilizations used storage cists.

GO ON TO THE NEXT PAGE.

Passage II (Questions 6 - 11)

It is a curious fact that in Assyria the ruins speak to us only of the living, and that of the dead there are no traces whatever. One might think people never died there at all. Yet it is well known that all nations have bestowed as much care on the interment of their dead and the adornment of their last resting-place as on the construction of their dwellings… some even more, for instance, the Egyptians. To this loving veneration for the dead history owes half its discoveries; indeed we should have almost no reliable information at all on the very oldest races, who lived before the invention of writing, were it not for their tombs and the things we find in them. It is very strange, therefore, that nothing of the kind should be found in Assyria, a country which stood so high in culture.

For the sepulchers which are found in such numbers in some mounds down to a certain depth, belong, as is shown by their very position, to later races, mostly even to the modern Turks and Arabs. This peculiarity is so puzzling that scholars almost incline to suppose that the Assyrians either made away with their dead in some manner unknown to us, or else took them somewhere to bury. The latter conjecture, though not entirely devoid of foundation, as we shall see, is unsupported by any positive facts, and therefore was never seriously discussed.

It is just the contrary in Babylonia. It can boast few handsome ruins or sculptures. The platforms and main walls of many palaces and temples have been known from the names stamped on the bricks and the cylinders found in the foundations, but they present only shapeless masses, from which all traces of artistic work have disappeared. In compensation, there is no country in the world where so many and such vast cemeteries have been discovered. It appears that the land of Chaldea,—perhaps because it was the cradle of nations which afterwards grew to greatness, as the Assyrians and the Hebrews—was regarded as a place of peculiar holiness by its own inhabitants, and probably also by neighboring countries, which would explain the mania that seems to have prevailed through so many ages, for burying the dead there in unheard of numbers. Strangely enough, some portions of it even now are held sacred in the same sense.

Among the Chaldeans cities Erech (now Warka) was considered from very old times one of the holiest. It had many extremely ancient temples and a college of learned priests, and around it gradually formed an immense "city of the dead" or Necropolis. The English explorer, Loftus, in 1854-5, specially turned his attention to it and his account is astounding. First of all, he was struck by the majestic desolation of the place. Warka and a few other mounds are raised on a slightly elevated tract of the desert, above the level of the yearly inundations, and accessible only from November to March… "The desolation and solitude of Warka," says Loftus, "are even more striking than the scene which is presented at Babylon itself. There is no life for miles around. No river glides in grandeur at the base of its mounds; no green date groves flourish near its ruins."

6. Which of the following statements is inconsistent with information in the passage?

A. Chaldea contained famous places of holiness.
B. European explorers visited Erech.
C. The dead were confiscated from Assyrian cities.
D. A very large site of buried citizens is sometimes referred to as a Necropolis.

GO ON TO THE NEXT PAGE.

7. Which of the following inferences is justified by information in the passage?

A. Chaldean cities became a Necropolis.
B. The Egyptians buried their dead in pots.
C. Temples of Babylonia suffered considerable damage.
D. Some regions of Chaldea are submerged under swamps in May.

8. The author of the passage probably most strongly supports:

A. proper burial of the dead.
B. logical arguments supported by evidence.
C. places of holiness.
D. written history.

9. If information in the passage is accurate, which of the following would one LEAST expect to find in ancient Assyria?

A. Empty tombs.
B. Greatly decorated final resting places that are intricately designed.
C. Temples of shapeless masses.
D. Designated locations of buried precious metals.

10. The author apparently believes that burial of the dead in great numbers in a single region is:

A. odd, especially if continued to present day.
B. not surprising if done using sepulchers.
C. correlated with the degree of holiness of an ancient city.
D. expected in civilizations high in culture.

11. Several cities and civilizations cited in the passage revealed unexpected findings EXCEPT for:

A. modern Turkey.
B. Warka.
C. Assyria.
D. Chaldea.

GO ON TO THE NEXT PAGE.

Passage III (Questions 12 - 18)

A common defect in standing timber results from radial splits which extend inward from the periphery of the tree, and almost, if not always, near the base. It is most common in trees which split readily, and those with large rays and thin bark. The primary cause of the splitting is frost, and various theories have been advanced to explain the action.

Hartig believes that freezing forces out a part of the… water of the cell walls, thereby causing the wood to shrink, and if the interior layers have not yet been cooled, tangential strains arise which finally produce radial clefts.

Another theory holds that the water is not driven out of the cell walls, but that difference in temperature conditions of inner and outer layers is itself sufficient to set up the strains, resulting in splitting. An air temperature of 14°F or less is considered necessary to produce frost splits.

A still more recent theory is that of Busse who considers the mechanical action of the wind a very important factor. He observed: (a) Frost splits sometimes occur at higher temperatures than 14°F; (b) Most splits take place shortly before sunrise, i.e., at the time of lowest air and soil temperature; they are never heard to take place at noon, afternoon, or evening; (c) They always occur between two roots or between the collars of two roots; (d) They are most frequent in old, stout-rooted, broad-crowned trees; in younger stands it is always the stoutest members that are found with frost splits, while in quite young stands they are altogether absent; (e) Trees on wet sites are most liable to splits, due to difference in wood structure, just as difference in wood structure makes different species vary in this regard; (f) Frost splits are most numerous within three feet of the ground.

When a tree is swayed by the wind the roots are counteracting forces, and the wood fibers are tested in tension and compression by the opposing forces; where the roots exercise tension stresses most effectively the effect of compression stresses is at a minimum; only where the pressure is in excess of the tension, i.e., between the roots, can a separation of the fiber result. Hence, when by frost a tension on the entire periphery is established, and the wind localizes additional strains, failure occurs. The stronger the compression and tension, the severer the strains and the oftener failures occur.

Heart shake occurs in nearly all overmature timber, being more frequent in hardwoods (especially oak) than in conifers. In typical heart shake the center of the hole shows indications of becoming hollow and radial clefts of varying size extend outward from the pith, being widest inward. It frequently affects only the butt log, but may extend to the entire hole and even the larger branches. It usually results from a shrinkage of the heartwood due probably to chemical changes in the wood.

When it consists of a single cleft extending across the pith it is termed simple heart shake. Shake of this character in straight-grained trees affects only one or two central boards when cut into lumber, but in spiral-grained timber the damage is much greater. When shake consists of several radial clefts it is termed star shake. In some instances one or more of these clefts may extend nearly to the bark. In felled or converted timber clefts due to heart shake may be distinguished from seasoning cracks by the darker color of the exposed surfaces. Such clefts, however, tend to open up more and more as the timber seasons.

12. It can most justifiably be said that the main purpose of the passage is:

A. to describe defensible theories of timber splits and shakes.
B. to clarify the principles of freezing wood.
C. to outline an analysis of tree damage.
D. to evaluate mechanisms of frost damage.

GO ON TO THE NEXT PAGE.

13. According to the passage, simple heart shake causes primarily which of the following forms of damage?

A. One cleft across the pith.
B. A hollow hole with radial clefts.
C. Several radial clefts.
D. A cleft across one or two boards of spiral grained timber.

14. The author of the passage would be most likely to agree with which of the following ideas?

A. Radial splits extend inward and usually near the middle trunk.
B. Without cold temperatures, splits do not occur.
C. The chemical nature of wood changes over time.
D. Splits are more common than shakes.

15. Suppose splits occurred on an old tree during a day of no wind. Busse would support which of the following statements as the most likely explanation?

A. The temperature rose above 14°F.
B. The frost alone produced enough tension to open old frost splits.
C. Wet sites produced condensation inside the cell walls of the tree.
D. Freezing forced out water from the cell walls.

16. On the basis of the passage, lighter-colored clefts in a converted hardwood that maintains its size over time is best described as:

A. Radial splits.
B. Star shake.
C. Seasoning cracks.
D. Heart shake.

17. Which of the following statements, if true, would most directly challenge the mechanical theory of radial splits?

A. Freezing forces water into cell walls.
B. Tension is always in excess of pressure.
C. Difference in temperature between inner and outer layers is insufficient to set up strains.
D. Most splits take place after sunrise.

18. Elsewhere, the author of the passage states that ring shake results from the concentric as well as radial shrinkage of heartwood. Ring shake may occur in connection with what other form of damage?

A. Frost splits.
B. Radial splits.
C. Log shake.
D. Heart shake.

GO ON TO THE NEXT PAGE.

Passage IV (Questions 19 - 24)

"Don't be so particular" is a particularly popular phrase. It comes up constantly from the rough quarry of human nature—is a part of life's untamed protest against punctiliousness and mathematical virtue. Particular people are never very popular people, just because they are particular…

…But it does not follow, etymologically, that a man is right because he is particular. He may be very good or very bad, and yet be only such because he is particularly so. Singularity, eccentricity, speciality, isolation, oddity, and hundreds of other things which might be mentioned, all involve particularity. But we do not intend, to "grammar-out" the question, nor to disengage and waste our gas in definitions.

The particular enters into all sorts of things, and it has even a local habitation and a name in religion. What could be more particular than Particular Baptism? Certain followers of a man belonging to the great Smith family constituted the first congregation of English Baptists. These were of the General type. The Particular Baptists trace their origin to a coterie of men and women who had an idea that their grace was of a special type…

The doctrines of the Particular Baptists are of the Calvinistic hue. They believe in eternal election, free justification, ultimate glorification; they have a firm notion that they are a special people, known before all time; that not one of them will be lost; and they differ from the General Baptists, so far as discipline is concerned, in this—they reject "open communion," will allow no membership prior to dipping; or,—to quote the exact words of one of them, who wrote to us the other day on the subject, and who paled our ineffectual fire very considerably with his definition—"All who enter our pail must be baptized." If there is any water in the "pail" they will; if not, it will be a simple question of dryness.

There is a great deal of heathenish contentment in Vauxhall-road district… The interior of Vauxhall-road Particular Baptist Chapel is specially plain and quiet looking, has nothing ornamental in it and at present having been newly cleaned, it smells more of paint than of anything else. The pews are of various dimensions— some long, some square, all high… This is not intended as a reflection upon the occupants, but is done as a simple matter of taste. The "members" of the chapel at present are neither increasing nor decreasing—are stationary…

Either the chapel is too near the street, or the street too near the chapel, or the children in the neighborhood too numerous and noisy; for on Sundays, mainly during the latter part of the day, there is an incessant, half-shouting, half-singing din, from troops of youngsters adjoining, who play all sorts of chorusing games, which must seriously annoy the worshippers.

The hymn books used contain, principally, pieces selected by the celebrated William Gadsby, and nobody in the chapel need ever be harassed for either length or variety of spiritual verse. They have above 1,100 hymns to choose from, and in length these hymns range from three to twenty-three verses.

Whilst inspecting one of the books recently we came to a hymn of thirteen verses, and thought that wasn't so bad—was partly long enough for anybody; but we grew suddenly pale on directly afterwards finding one nearly twice the size—one with twenty-three mortal verses in it. It is to be hoped the choir and the congregation will never he called upon to sing right through any hymn extending to that disheartening and elastic length. We have heard a chapel choir sing a hymn of twelve verses, and felt ready for a stimulant afterwards to revive our exhausted energies; if twenty-three verses had to be fought through at one standing, in our hearing, we should smile with a musical ghastliness and perish.

GO ON TO THE NEXT PAGE.

19. According to the passage, a Particular Baptist would agree with each of the following tenets EXCEPT for:

A. justification.
B. being particular.
C. open communion.
D. baptism.

20. Suppose that the Particular Baptist Chapel were moved further away from the street. The most likely result of this action would be that:

A. Services would be held earlier in the mornings.
B. Calvinist membership would decrease.
C. Fewer children would attend church.
D. Membership would increase.

21. Which of the following findings, if true, would suggest that the author's concern about unpleasant experiences is exaggerated?

A. The congregations are encouraged by elevated volumes.
B. People living in the Vauxhall-road district stop attending church.
C. Baptists convert to a different religion en masse.
D. Members of the Baptist Chapel ceased singing hymns in church.

22. On the basis of information in the passage, one would generally expect the members of Vauxhall-road Particular Baptist Chapel to be:

A. pious.
B. frugal.
C. austere.
D. quiet.

23. The example of the General Baptists is most relevant to the author's assertion that particular people in a religion:

A. risk going too far to the detriment of its own members.
B. miss opportunities to challenge their own thinking.
C. trap themselves by becoming too rigid.
D. are actually more particular than members of the Particular Baptists.

24. The author would question which of the following statements:

A. Calvinists are just as strict as Baptists.
B. Unpopular people might be very particular.
C. A handful of concepts involve particularity.
D. The various ways in which people decorate a building reflect more their tastes than their judgments.

GO ON TO THE NEXT PAGE.

Passage V (Questions 25 - 29)

The calumet, or pipe of peace, ornamented with the war eagles quill, is a sacred pipe, and never used on any other occasion than that of peace making, when the chief brings it into treaty, and unfolding the many bandages which are carefully kept around it, has it ready to be mutually smoked by the chiefs, after the terms of the treaty are agreed upon, as the means of solemnizing it; which is done by passing the sacred stem to each chief, who draws one breath of smoke only through it. Nothing can be more binding than smoking the pipe of peace and is considered by them to be an inviolable pledge.

There is no custom more uniformly in constant use amongst the poor [Native Americans] than that of smoking nor any more highly valued. His pipe is his constant companion through life—his messenger of peace; he pledges his friends through its stem and its bowl, and when its care-drowning fumes cease to flow, it takes a place with him in his solitary grave with his tomahawk and war-club companions to his long-fancied happy hunting grounds.

The tobacco plant seems to have been cultivated in Mexico from time immemorial. Francisco Lopez de Gomara, who was chaplain to Cortez, when he made conquest of Mexico, in 1519, alludes to the plant and the custom of smoking; and Diaz relates that the king Montezuma had his pipe brought with much ceremony by the chief ladies of his court, after he had dined and washed his mouth with scented water.

The Spaniards encouraged its cultivation, and to this day it is grown in several of the coast states. Various kinds are cultivated, but chiefly a variety bearing yellow flowers, with a large leaf of fine flavor resembling the Havana. The plant is a favorite with the Mexicans, who prefer it to any other product grown. It is cultivated like most varieties of the tropics, and is hardly inferior to any grown in the West Indies, and is especially adapted for cigars and cigaritos. After the first harvest another, and sometimes a third crop is gathered by allowing one shoot to grow from the parent root, which oftentimes develops to a considerable size. The quality of leaf, however, is inferior; as is the case with all second and third crops grown in this manner.

The smoking of cigars is now considered the best as it is the most fashionable mode of using the weed. The word cigar is from the Spanish cigarro, and signifies a cylindrical roll of tobacco leaves, made of short pieces or shreds of the leaves divested of the stem and wound about with a binder, and enveloped in a portion of the leaf known by the name of wrapper—acute at one end and truncated at the other.

In the East Indies a sort of cigar called cheroot is also made with both ends truncated. The smoking of tobacco in the form of cigars is doubtless the most general as well as the most ancient mode of its use. When Columbus landed in Hispaniola, the sailors saw the natives smoking the leaves of a plant, "the perfume of which was fragrant and grateful."

In London the Yara is a favorite with many old smokers, who use no others. Old smokers describe the Yara cigar as having a "sweet" flavor, but one unaccustomed to them, like Hazard and others, pronounce them bitter, and having a "peculiar saline taste." It can, doubtless, be said with truth concerning the Yara cigar, that unlike other varieties, such as Havana, Manila, Paraguayan, Swiss and Brazil, the taste for them is not natural, but, when once formed, becomes very decided. As a general rule smokers of Yara cigars think other kinds are deficient in flavor, and are wanting in quality, because they lack the peculiar flavor belonging only to Yara cigars.

GO ON TO THE NEXT PAGE.

25. The assertion that tobacco has been cultivated in Mexico "from time immemorial" is:

A. contradicted by the assertion that the Spaniards introduced the plant to Mexico.
B. possibly true but not supported by examples or evidence.
C. true, given the findings of explorers.
D. supported by objective data in the passage.

26. One can justifiably infer from the author's comments about tobacco that there exists:

A. various kinds of plant, each with a distinct taste.
B. dozens of kinds of plants.
C. generations of crops of superior quality.
D. wealthy merchants in the business of selling tobacco products.

27. Which of the following statements captures the sentiments of the author the LEAST?

A. The earliest use of tobacco was in the form of cigars.
B. Without a doubt the Yara has an unnatural taste.
C. People tend to appreciate one taste to the point of disliking other tastes.
D. Tobacco was highly valued, but not ubiquitously used among Native Americans.

28. The author would most likely disagree with which of the following statements about tobacco:

A. Natives of Central America used tobacco in the form of cigars.
B. In general, tobacco products have a pleasing flavor.
C. Cigars are made by using a binder, and truncating one end.
D. Overall, tobacco products from Manilla are as high in quality as those from Havana, and even London.

29. Which of the following examples in the passage regarding various uses of tobacco demonstrates irony?

A. The predilection of Londoners to smoke the Yara.
B. The post-dinner ceremonies of king Montezuma.
C. The burial rituals of Native Americans.
D. The discoveries made by Columbus and Lopez de Gomara.

———————————————

GO ON TO THE NEXT PAGE.

Passage VI (Questions 30 - 34)

There is no cookery in Europe so often maligned without cause as that of Italy. People who are not sure of their facts often dismiss it contemptuously as being "all garlic and oil," whereas very little oil is used except at Genoa, where oil, and very good oil as a rule, takes the place of butter, and no more garlic than is necessary to give a slight flavor to the dishes in which it plays a part. An Italian cook fries better than one of any other nationality.

In the north very good meat is obtainable, the boiled beef of Turin being almost equal to our own Silverside. Farther and farther south, as the climate becomes hotter, the meat becomes less and less the food of the people, various dishes of pasta and fish taking its place, and as a compensation the fruit and the wine become more delicious. The fowls and figs of Tuscany, the white truffles of Piedmont, the artichokes of Rome, the walnuts and grapes of Sorrento, might well stir a gourmet to poetic flights.

Switzerland is a country of hotels and not of restaurants. In most of the big towns the hotels have restaurants attached to them, and in some of these a dinner ordered à la carte is just as well cooked as in a good French restaurant, and served as well; in other restaurants attached to good hotels the table-d'hôte dinner is served at separate tables at any time between certain hours, and this is the custom of most of the restaurants in most of the better class of hotels.

There is in every little mountain-hotel a restaurant; but this is generally used only by invalids, or very proud persons, or mountaineers coming back late from a climb. There is no country in which the gourmet has to adapt himself so much to circumstances and in which he does it, thanks to exercise and mountain air, with such a Chesterfieldian grace.

A candid Frenchman, who had lived long in Spain, asked as to the cookery of Spain compared with that of other nations, replied, "It is worse even than that of the English, which is the next worst." That Frenchman was, however, rather ungrateful, for the Spaniards taught the French how to stuff turkeys with chestnuts.

The Spanish cooks also first understood that an orange salad is the proper accompaniment to a wild duck, and the Spanish hams are excellent. The lower orders in Spain have too great a partiality for ajo and aceite for oil and garlic. Their oil, which they use greatly even with fish, is not the refined oil of Genoa or the south of France, but is a coarse liquid, the ill taste of which remains all day in one's mouth. Garlic is an excellent seasoning in its proper place and quantity, and the upper classes of the Spaniards have their meat lightly rubbed with it before being cooked, but the lower classes use it in the cooking to an intolerable extent.

The cuisine of the best of the Viennese restaurants, those attached to the big hotels, is French, though the Wiener Rostbraten and the Wiener Schnitzel are world-famous, and the typical Viennese dinner is a good French dinner with the addition of very delicious bread and pastry made with a lighter hand than any Gallic cook brings to his task. The wines of the country of Retz, Mailberg, Pfaffstadt, Gumpoldskirchen, Klosterneuberg, Nussberg, and Vöslau should all be tasted, most of them being more than drinkable. Beer, however, is the real Viennese drink, and the very light liquid, ice cold, is a delightful beverage.

GO ON TO THE NEXT PAGE.

30. For which of the following conclusions does the passage offer the most support?

A. Switzerland has too few restaurants.
B. Colder climates favor fish as the main cuisine.
C. Italian cuisine tastes better than that of all other nations.
D. The poor tend to misuse ingredients.

31. Which cuisine suffers from the greatest amount of undeserved criticism?

A. Spanish.
B. Austrian.
C. Swiss.
D. Italian.

32. Which of the following decisions based on Italian cuisine, if true, would best serve as an example for the candid Frenchman if he were living in Italy?

A. Despite the very oily taste of Italian cuisine, the contributions of Sorrento walnuts to French cuisine should be recognized.
B. Despite the rumors that Italian cuisine is too oily, the contributions of Sorrento walnuts to French cuisine should be recognized.
C. Despite the very oily taste of Italian cuisine, the contributions of Sorrento walnuts to Spanish cuisine should be recognized.
D. Despite the rumors that Italian cuisine is too oily, the contributions of Sorrento walnuts to Spanish cuisine should be recognized.

33. Assume that a Frenchman gave a favorable critique of the cuisine in Switzerland. The author would most likely find this critique:

A. somewhat surprising since the French are the most critical of cuisine from other nations.
B. probable, given the quality of à la carte dinners in big towns.
C. remarkable, given the Frenchman's failure to realize Spain's contributions to French cuisine.
D. very surprising because Switzerland is a country of hotels and not of restaurants.

34. Suppose that the author could decide where to eat a dinner containing garlic and oil. Where would the author prefer to eat this meal?

A. Austria.
B. Spain.
C. Italy.
D. Switzerland.

_____

GO ON TO THE NEXT PAGE.

Passage VII (Questions 35 - 40)

Conspicuous in their myths is the tale of the Two Brothers. These mysterious beings are upon the earth before man appears. Though alone, they do not agree, and the one attacks and slays the other. Another brother appears on the scene, who seems to be the one slain, who has come to life, and the two are given wives by the Being who was the Creator of things. These two women were perfectly beautiful, but invisible to the eyes of mortals. The one was named, The Woman of the Light or The Woman of the Morning; the other was the Woman of Darkness or the Woman of Evening. The brothers lived together in one tent with these women, who each in turn went out to work. When the Woman of Light was at work, it was daytime; when the Woman of Darkness was at her labors, it was night.

In another myth of this stock, clearly a version of the former, this father of the race is represented as a mighty bird, called Yêl, or Yale, or Orelbale, from the root ell, a term they apply to everything supernatural. He took to wife the daughter of the Sun (the Woman of Light), and by her begat the race of man. He formed the dry land for a place for them to live upon, and stocked the rivers with salmon, that they might have food. When he enters his nest it is day, but when he leaves it is night; or, according to another myth, he has the two women for wives, the one of whom makes the day, the other the night.

Of course, the daily history of the appearance and disappearance of light is intimately connected with the apparent motion of the sun. Hence, in the myths there is often a seeming identification of the two, which I have been at no pains to avoid. But the identity is superficial only; it entirely disappears in other parts of the myth, and the conceptions, as fundamentally distinct, must be studied separately, to reach accurate results. It is an easy, but by no means a profound method of treating these religions, to dismiss them all by the facile explanations of "animism," and "sun and moon worship."

…I think that most modern ethnologists will agree that it is no more possible for races in all stages of culture and of widely different faculties to receive with benefit any one religion, than it is for them to thrive under one form of government, or to adopt with advantage one uniform plan of building houses. The moral and religious life is a growth, and the brash wood of ancient date cannot be grafted on the green stem. It is well to remember that the heathendoms of America were very far from wanting living seeds of sound morality and healthy mental education…

In their origin in the human mind, religion and morality have nothing in common. They are even antagonistic. At the root of all religions is the passionate desire for the widest possible life, for the most unlimited exercise of all the powers. The basis of all morality is self-sacrifice, the willingness to give up our wishes to the will of another. The criterion of the power of a religion is its ability to command this sacrifice; the criterion of the excellence of a religion is the extent to which its commands coincide with the good of the race, with the lofty standard of the "categorical imperative."

GO ON TO THE NEXT PAGE.

35. The author is primarily concerned with demonstrating that:

A. Morality serves the foundation for many cultures.
B. Religion is a complex entity that cannot be simplified.
C. Myths, like religions, are unpredictable.
D. Mythologies from different cultures share common themes.

36. The author describes women as representing each of the following EXCEPT:

A. goodness.
B. the invisible.
C. the mother of all mankind.
D. daylight.

37. The author would most likely agree with which of the following about religion?

A. The source of all religion is self sacrifice.
B. Religion and morality share a common purpose.
C. The female element plays a central theme in religions.
D. Animism lies at the heart of religion.

38. Which of the following, if true, would most *weaken* the author's argument?

A. Man has a basic desire for unlimited power.
B. Historical documents disprove the cultural imperative.
C. Archeologists discover religious texts describing mythological animals giving birth to all of mankind.
D. The basis of morality is hedonism.

39. The author states that "the brash wood of ancient date cannot be grafted on the green stem." The most likely purpose of this reference is to show that:

A. Old ideas cannot be imposed on younger generations.
B. Moral thought and religious life are a work-in-progress.
C. Many citizens do not desire a moral code.
D. Morality can undermine religion.

40. The word "heathendoms" most clearly represents:

A. Martyrs.
B. Philosophers.
C. Agnostics.
D. Renegades.

STOP.   IF YOU FINISH BEFORE TIME IS CALLED, CHECK YOUR WORK. YOU MAY GO BACK TO ANY QUESTION IN THIS TEST.

STOP.

Verbal Reasoning Test 2

Time: 60 Minutes
Questions 1 - 40

VERBAL REASONING

DIRECTIONS: There are seven passages in the Verbal Reasoning test. Each passage is followed by five to seven questions. Pace yourself and select the one best answer to each question.

Passage I (Questions 1 - 5)

At the creation of the world, lesser powers were made, because Tira'wa-tius, the Mighty Power, could not come near to man, or be seen or felt by him. These lesser powers dwell in the great circle of the sky. One is North Star; another is Brown Eagle. The Winds were the first of the lesser powers to come near man. Therefore, when man calls for aid, he calls first to the Winds. They stand at the four points, and guard the four paths down which the lesser powers come when they help mankind. The Winds are always near us, by day and by night.

The Sun is one of these powers. It comes from the mighty power above; therefore it has great strength. Mother Earth is another power. She is very near to man. From her we get food; upon her we lie down. We live and walk on her. We could not exist without Mother Earth, without Sun, and without the Winds.

Water is another lesser power. Water is necessary to mankind. Fire made by rubbing two sticks together is sacred. It comes direct from the power granted Toharu, vegetation, in answer to man's prayer as he rubs the sticks. When the flame leaps from the glowing wood, it is the word of the fire. The power has come near.
Blue is the color of the sky, the dwelling place of Tira´wahut, the circle of powers which watch over man. As a man paints the blue stick he sings.

Red is the color of the sun. Green is the color of Mother Earth.

Eagle is the chief of day; Owl is chief of the night; Woodpecker is chief of the trees; Duck is chief of the water.

The ear of corn represents the supernatural power that dwells in the earth, which brings forth the food that sustains life; there corn is spoken of as h'Atira, "mother breathing forth life." The power which dwells in the earth, which enables it to give life to all growing things, comes from above. Therefore, in the Hako, the Pawnee ceremony, the ear of corn is painted with blue.

The wildcat was made to live in the forest. He has much skill and ingenuity. The wildcat shows us we must think, must use tact, must be shrewd when we set out to do anything. The wildcat is one of the sacred animals. Trees grow along the banks of the streams; we can see them at a distance, like a long line, and we can see the river glistening in the sunlight in its length. We sing to the river, and when we come nearer and see the water and hear it rippling along, then we sing to the water, the water that ripples as it runs.

Hills were made by Tira'wa. We ascend hills when we go away alone to pray. From the top of a hill we can look over the country to see if there are enemies in sight, or if any danger is near us. We can see if we are to meet friends. The hills help man, so we sing to them.

GO ON TO THE NEXT PAGE.

1. The passage implies that a man who does not sing as he paints with a blue stick probably:

A. does not believe that Tira´ wahut can help him.
B. believes Toharu can help him instead.
C. does so out of respect for the sky.
D. is appealing to the lesser power of Silence.

2. According to the passage, each of the following lesser powers come down to help mankind EXCEPT:

A. Brown Eagle.
B. Sun.
C. North Star.
D. Winds.

3. Suppose that the Pawnee believed that the Ox represents the power which brings forth fighting strength, and that this power comes from the night. In the Hako, fighting power would most likely be represented by:

A. the Ox with an Owl painted on it.
B. the Ox painted with black.
C. the Owl painted with blue.
D. the Owl with an Ox painted on it.

4. According to the passage, the Pawnee would interpret the flame from a burning stick to be:

A. Sun speaking, since fire comes from the Sun.
B. Mother Earth speaking, since all life comes from her.
C. Wood speaking, in answer to man's prayer.
D. Fire speaking, with permission from Toharu.

5. Suppose that Water was the first of the lesser powers to come near man. How would this impact man's call for aid?

A. Man would make sure to live by a body of water.
B. Water would become the source of all lesser powers.
C. Man would still call to the Winds first, since they are always near him.
D. Man could not call for aid because the Winds would be a lesser power.

GO ON TO THE NEXT PAGE.

Passage II (Question 6 - 11)

It follows that since Germany manufactures so well at home, she diminishes her imports from France and England year by year. She has not only become their rival in manufactured goods in Asia and in Africa, but also in London and in Paris. Shortsighted people in France may cry out against the Frankfort Treaty; English manufacturers may explain German competition by little differences in railway tariffs; they may linger on the petty side of questions, and neglect great historical facts. But it is none the less certain that the main industries, formerly in the hands of England and France, have progressed eastward, and in Germany they have found a country, young, full of energy, possessing an intelligent middle class, and eager in its turn to enrich itself by foreign trade.

Economists hold the customs responsible for these facts, and yet cottons manufactured in Russia are sold at the same price as in London. Capital taking no cognizance of father-lands, German and English capitalists, accompanied by engineers and foremen of their own nationalities, have introduced in Russia and in Poland manufactories whose goods compete in excellence with the best from England. If customs were abolished to-morrow, manufacture would only gain by it. Not long ago the British manufacturers delivered another hard blow to the import of cloth and woolens from the West. They set up in southern and middle Russia immense wool factories, stocked with the most perfect machinery from Bradford, and already now Russia imports only the highest sorts of cloth and woolen fabrics from England, France and Austria. The remainder is fabricated at home, both in factories and as domestic industries.

We all know the theory: the great European nations need colonies, for colonies send raw material—cotton fiber, unwashed wool, spices, etc., to the mother-land. And the mother-land, under pretense of sending them manufactured wares, gets rid of her damaged stuffs, her machine scrap-iron and everything which she no longer has any use for. It costs her little or nothing, and none the less the articles are sold at exorbitant prices.

Such was the theory—such was the practice for a long time. In London and Manchester fortunes were made, while India was being ruined. In the India Museum in London unheard of riches, collected in Calcutta and Bombay by English merchants, are to be seen.

But other English merchants and capitalists conceived the very simple idea that it would be more expedient to exploit the natives of India by making cotton-cloth in India itself, than to import from twenty to twenty-four million pounds' worth of goods annually.

At first a series of experiments ended in failure. Indian weavers—artists and experts in their own craft—could not inure themselves to factory life; the machinery sent from Liverpool was bad; the climate had to be taken into account; and merchants had to adapt themselves to new conditions, now fully mastered, before British India could become the menacing rival of the Mother-land she is to-day.

And why should India not manufacture? What should be the hindrance? Capital?—But capital goes wherever there are men, poor enough to be exploited. Knowledge? But knowledge recognizes no national barriers. Technical skill of the worker?—No. Are, then, Hindu workmen inferior to the hundreds of thousands of boys and girls, not eighteen years old, at present working in the English textile factories?

GO ON TO THE NEXT PAGE.

6. According to the author, what is the main factor that regulated the economy in the twentieth century?

A. Prices of imports from India.
B. Manufacturing in Russia, India, and Germany.
C. Cheap labor beyond the shores of England.
D. Colonies competing with the mother-land in their production of manufactured goods.

7. According to the passage, the business exploits of England merchants in India:

A. Suffered from a clash of cultures.
B. Struggled to understand the needs of workers in India.
C. Lost profit from broken machinery.
D. Succeeded initially, but then succumbed to the failures of machinery and climate.

8. With which of the following opinions would the author most likely *disagree*?

A. India is a country that should manufacture goods.
B. Countries with cheap labor are limited by capital.
C. Laborers in industrialized nations are as skilled as workers in less developed countries.
D. Business practices of English colonization evolved into a more exploitative power.

9. The example of Germany serves primarily to:

A. Explain the natural progression of industrious nations becoming economically independent.
B. Highlight the inferior manufacturing of France and England.
C. Emphasize the growing competition faced by English manufacturing.
D. Give proof against the specialization of national industry.

10. Suppose that a once-agricultural country such as Brazil evolved to become a manufacturing power of cotton. The author would most likely find this news to be:

A. a notable exception.
B. not surprising.
C. expected.
D. not possible given the theory of colonization.

11. Suppose that a tax on imported Russian goods into England were abolished. The most likely outcome of this action would be:

A. Sales of British goods in Russia would increase.
B. Sales of Russian goods in Russia would increase.
C. Sales of British goods in England would decrease.
D. No change due to the inferior quality of Russian goods.

_____

GO ON TO THE NEXT PAGE.

Passage III (Questions 12 - 16)

At the time of the overthrow of the Shang and establishment of the Chou dynasty in 1122 B.C. there lived two marshals, Chêng Lung and Ch'ên Ch'i. These were Hêng and Ha, the Snorter and Blower respectively. The former was the chief superintendent of supplies for the armies of the tyrant emperor Chou, the Nero of China. The latter was in charge of the victualling department of the same army.

From his master, Tu O, the celebrated Taoist magician of the K'un-lun Mountains, Hêng acquired a marvellous power. When he snorted, his nostrils, with a sound like that of a bell, emitted two white columns of light, which destroyed his enemies, body and soul. Thus through him the Chou gained numerous victories… Later on he found himself face to face with the Blower. The latter had learnt from the magician how to store in his chest a supply of yellow gas which, when he blew it out, annihilated anyone whom it struck. By this means he caused large gaps to be made in the ranks of the enemy.

Being opposed to each other, the one snorting out great streaks of white light, the other blowing streams of yellow gas, the combat continued until the Blower was wounded in the shoulder by No-cha, of the army of Chou, and pierced in the stomach with a spear by Huang Fei-hu, Yellow Flying Tiger…

The functions discharged by Hêng and Ha at the gates of Buddhist temples are in Taoist temples discharged by Blue Dragon and White Tiger.

The former, the Spirit of the Blue Dragon Star, was Têng Chiu-kung, one of the chief generals of the last emperor of the Yin dynasty. He had a son named Têng Hsiu, and a daughter named Ch'an-yü.

The army of Têng Chiu-kung was camped at San-shan Kuan, when he received orders to proceed to the battle then taking place at Hsi Ch'i. There, in standing up to No-cha and Huang Fei-hu, he had his left arm broken by the former's magic bracelet, but, fortunately

for him, his subordinate, T'u Hsing-sun, a renowned magician, gave him a remedy which quickly healed the fracture.

His daughter then came on the scene to avenge her father. She had a magic weapon, the Five-fire Stone, which she hurled full in the face of Yang Chien. But the Immortal was not wounded; on the other hand, his celestial dog jumped at Ch'an-yü and bit her neck, so that she was obliged to flee. T'u Hsing-sun, however, healed the wound.

After a banquet, Têng Chiu-kung promised his daughter in marriage to T'u Hsing-sun if he would gain him the victory at Hsi Ch'i. Chiang Tzŭ-ya then persuaded T'u's magic master, Chü Liu-sun, to call his disciple over to his camp, where he asked him why he was fighting against the new dynasty. "Because," he replied, "Chiu-kung has promised me his daughter in marriage as a reward of success." Chiang Tzŭ-ya thereupon promised to obtain the bride, and sent a force to seize her. As a result of the fighting that ensued, Chiu-kung was beaten, and retreated in confusion, leaving Ch'an-yü in the hands of the victors. During the next few days the marriage was celebrated with great ceremony in the victor's camp. According to custom, the bride returned for some days to her father's house, and while there she earnestly exhorted Chiu-kung to submit. Following her advice, he went over to Chiang Tzŭ-ya's party.

In the ensuing battles he fought valiantly on the side of his former enemy, and killed many famous warriors, but he was eventually attacked by the Blower, from whose mouth a column of yellow gas struck him, throwing him from his steed…

GO ON TO THE NEXT PAGE.

12. Which of the following events, references, or ideas does not appear in the passage?

A. An astrological figure.
B. A Roman general.
C. A magical boy.
D. A military retreat.

13. The passage suggests that Têng Chiu-kung most likely felt:

A. proud of Ch'an-yü.
B. betrayed by T'u Hsing-sun.
C. cautious about Chü Liu-sun.
D. approval of Têng Hsiu.

14. Conflict between each of the following pairs is depicted in the passage EXCEPT between:

A. the Chou Dynasty and Yin Dynasty.
B. the Yellow Flying Tiger and the Blower.
C. the Blue Dragon and the Chou Dynasty.
D. the Snorter and the Blue Dragon.

15. According to the passage, Têng Chiu-kung fought on the side of:

A. the Yin Dynasty.
B. the Chou Dynasty.
C. both the Yin and Chou Dynasties.
D. neither the Yin nor Chou Dynasties.

16. The passage depicts the columns of light of the Snorter, and the yellow gas of the Blower. This is a reflection of:

A. an author attempting to add a sense of immortality to venerated Chinese military generals.
B. factual military leaders who served in the ancient Chinese army.
C. an author staying true to Chinese folklore.
D. ancient Chinese fiction.

GO ON TO THE NEXT PAGE.

Passage IV (Questions 17 - 21)

Man is not a being whose exclusive purpose in life is eating, drinking, and providing a shelter for himself. As soon as his material wants are satisfied, other needs, which, generally speaking, may be described as of an artistic character, will thrust themselves forward. These needs are of the greatest variety; they vary with each and every individual; and the more society is civilized, the more will individuality be developed, and the more will desires be varied.

Even to-day we see men and women denying themselves necessaries to acquire mere trifles, to obtain some particular gratification, or some intellectual or material enjoyment… Would life, with all its inevitable drudge and sorrows, be worth living, if, besides daily work, man could never obtain a single pleasure according to his individual tastes?

If we wish for a Social Revolution, it is no doubt, first of all, to give bread to everyone; to transform this execrable society, in which we can every day see capable workmen dangling their arms for want of an employer who will exploit them; women and children wandering shelterless at night; whole families reduced to dry bread; men, women, and children dying for want of care and even for want of food. It is to put an end to these iniquities that we rebel.

But we expect more from the Revolution. We see that the worker, compelled to struggle painfully for bare existence, is reduced to ignore the higher delights, the highest within man's reach, of science, and especially of scientific discovery; of art, and especially of artistic creation. It is in order to obtain for all of us joys that are now reserved to a few; in order to give leisure and the possibility of developing everyone's intellectual capacities, that the social revolution must guarantee daily bread to all. After bread has been secured, leisure is the supreme aim.

Everybody does not need a telescope, because, even if learning were general, there are people who prefer to examine things through a microscope to studying the starry heavens. Some like statues, some like pictures. A particular individual has no other ambition than to possess a good piano, while another is pleased with an accordion… Still he cherishes the hope of some day satisfying his tastes more or less, and for this reason he reproaches the idealist Communist societies with having the material life of each individual as their sole aim. "In your communal stores you may perhaps have bread for all," he says to us, "but you will not have beautiful pictures, optical instruments, luxurious furniture, artistic jewelry—in short, the many things that minister to the infinite variety of human tastes…"

These are the objections which all communist systems have to consider, and which the founders of new societies, established in American deserts, never understood. They believed that if the community could procure sufficient cloth to dress all its members, a music-room in which the "brothers" could strum a piece of music, or act a play from time to time, it was enough… In vain did the community guarantee the common necessaries of life, in vain did it suppress all education that would tend to develop individuality… The society could only exist on condition that it crushed all individual feeling, all artistic tendency, and all development.

Will the anarchist Commune be impelled by the same direction?—Evidently not, if it understands that while it produces all that is necessary to material life, it must also strive to satisfy all manifestations of the human mind.

GO ON TO THE NEXT PAGE.

17. Which of the following discoveries, if true, would most *weaken* the author's argument?

A. An anarchist Commune that feeds and clothes all of its members.
B. A Communist society in which each member owns a scientific instrument.
C. A social revolution that guarantees daily bread for all.
D. A free society that engages in a revolution and becomes Communist.

18. Each of the following statements is supported by the passage EXCEPT:

A. Tastes vary, but artistic needs exist in all.
B. Some citizens like statues, while others like pictures.
C. Clothing all members is sufficient for a society to exist.
D. The exploitation of labor is not uncommon.

19. The passage addresses an important relationship between:

A. Leisure and the success of the social revolution.
B. Luxury and the fall of the anarchist Commune.
C. Freedom and the fall of the Communist system.
D. Work and the hope of luxury.

20. According to the passage, which of the following is most likely true about the relationship between inner need and society?

A. Each citizen is guided by the same fundamental desires.
B. The more civilized a society, the more time its citizens will have to enjoy more luxuries.
C. An uncivilized society does not have to meet as many needs as an advanced society.
D. The members of an anarchy will have the greatest variety of needs.

21. According to one historical authority on the idealist Communist society, "…you suppress the possibility of obtaining anything besides the bread and meat which the commune can offer to all, and the drab linen in which all your lady citizens will be dressed." The authority would probably:

A. Agree with the author's beliefs about the social revolution.
B. Support the main critics of the author.
C. Caution the founders of idealist societies.
D. Object to the author's claim about anarchist Communes.

GO ON TO THE NEXT PAGE.

Passage V (Questions 22 - 28)

As to disease, it is so rare in wild animals, or in a large majority of cases so quickly proves fatal, that, compared with what we call disease in our own species it is practically non-existent. The "struggle for existence," in so far as animals in a state of nature are concerned, is a metaphorical struggle; and the strife, short and sharp, which is so common in nature, is not misery, although it results in pain, since it is pain that kills or is soon outlived.

Fear there is, just as in fine weather there are clouds in the sky; and just as the shadow of the cloud passes, so does fear pass from the wild creature when the object that excited it has vanished from sight. And when death comes, it comes unexpectedly, and is not the death that we know, even before we taste of it, thinking of it with apprehension all our lives long, but a sudden blow that takes away consciousness—the touch of something that numbs the nerves—merely the prick of a needle.

In whatever way the animal perishes, whether by violence, or excessive cold, or decay, his death is a comparatively easy one. So long as he is fighting with or struggling to escape from an enemy, wounds are not felt as wounds, and scarcely hurt him—as we know from our own experience; and when overcome, if death be not practically instantaneous, as in the case of a small bird seized by a cat, the disabling grip or blow is itself a kind of anodyne, producing insensibility to pain.

This, too, is a matter of human experience. To say nothing of those who fall in battle, men have often been struck down and fearfully lacerated by lions, tigers, jaguars, and other savage beasts; and after having been rescued by their companions, have recounted this strange thing. Even when there was no loss of consciousness, when they saw and knew that the animal was rending their flesh, they seemed not to feel it, and were, at the time, indifferent to the fate that had overtaken them.

It is the same in death from cold. The strong, well-nourished man, overtaken by a snowstorm on some pathless, uninhabited waste, may experience some exceedingly bitter moments, or even hours, before he gives up the struggle. The physical pain is simply nothing: the whole bitterness is in the thought that he must die. The horror at the thought of annihilation, the remembrance of all the happiness he is now about to lose, of dear friends, of those whose lives will be dimmed with grief for his loss, of all his cherished dreams of the future—the sting of all this is so sharp that, compared with it, the creeping coldness in his blood is nothing more than a slight discomfort, and is scarcely felt. By and by he is overcome by drowsiness, and ceases to struggle… And when he sleeps he passes away; very easily, very painlessly, for the pain was of the mind, and was over long before death ensued.

The bird, however hard the frost may be, flies briskly to its customary roosting-place, and with beak tucked into its wing, falls asleep. It has no apprehensions; only the hot blood grows colder and colder, the pulse feebler as it sleeps, and at midnight, or in the early morning, it drops from its perch—dead.

Those of my readers who have seen much of animals in a state of nature, will agree that death from decay, or old age, is very rare among them. In that state the fullest vigor, with brightness of all the faculties, is so important that probably in ninety-nine cases in a hundred any falling-off in strength, or decay of any sense, results in some fatal accident. Death by misadventure, as we call it, is Nature's ordinance, the end designed for a very large majority of her children.

GO ON TO THE NEXT PAGE.

22. Which of the following circumstances would the author accept as a probable explanation for the one in a hundred animals that die from old age?

A. The animal possessed greater natural strength and stamina.
B. The animal was near the top of the food chain.
C. The animals was able to overcome all threats and attacks.
D. The creature was lucky enough to have never faced a fatal accident.

23. Implicit in the passage is the assumption that:

A. Dying is a peaceful process.
B. Animals are without much thought.
C. Humans accept death when it arrives.
D. Fear and death are separate entities.

24. An editor who is critical of the author would most likely support which of the following statements?

A. Pain is the final sensation before death.
B. Death from old age is very rare.
C. Physical pain from dying in cold is not significant.
D. Disease is rare in wild animals.

25. The author treats the ideas of death in animals and that in humans as distinct from each other. Which of the following characteristics supports this distinction?

A. Pain.
B. Fear.
C. Decay.
D. Survival.

26. According to the passage, which of the following circumstances describe a *difficult death*?

A. Two tigers attacking each other.
B. A soldier wounded by an enemy's blade.
C. A seal bleeding from a polar bear attack.
D. A deer pierced by a hunter's arrow.

27. What role does the idea of a cloud play in the passage?

A. It offers a symbol of calm that characterizes the nature of painless death.
B. It reminds the reader that the source of fear is not lasting.
C. It is a metaphor for fear.
D. It offers a representation of death.

28. The passage would most likely appear in which of the following formats?

A. A report in an anthropology journal.
B. An editorial in a zoology publication.
C. A philosophical treatise on dying.
D. A sociology journal.

GO ON TO THE NEXT PAGE.

Passage VI (Questions 29 - 34)

When a meter is used on a water system, the water company demands that a check valve be placed on the hot-water system to prevent the hot water from being forced back into the meter in case the pressure got strong enough in the boiler. If a check valve is used for this purpose, or for any other purpose, a safety valve must be placed on the boiler piping system to relieve any excessive pressure that may be caused by having the check valve in use. There is today, with meters of modern type, no reason to use a check valve or a safety valve. If an excessive pressure is obtained in the boiler, it is relieved in the water main.

When water is heated, it expands. If the heat becomes more intense and steam is formed, the expansion is much greater, and some means must be provided to allow for it. This expansion can be allowed to relieve itself in the water main as explained above. When a check valve is placed on the piping, this means of escape is shut off and a safety valve must be employed. Without these reliefs, the pressure would be so great that an explosion would result. When steel pipe and steel boilers are used for storage tanks and connections, the pipe and tank will shortly start to rust and parts of the piping are stopped up with rust scales. The water also becomes red with rust when the water becomes hot enough to circulate. When the pipes are stopped up, steam is formed and a snapping and cracking sound is heard.

To avoid these conditions, the piping should be of brass or lead and the storage tank should be of copper. The installation cost of brass and copper is greater than steel, but they will not have to be replaced in two or three years, as is the case with other material. A valve should be placed on the cold-water supply to control the entire hot-water piping system. A pipe with a stop cock should be placed underneath the boiler and should extend into a sink in the basement so that the boiler can be drained at any time for cleaning or repairs.

First of all, the covering must be put on properly to be of high service. Hot-water circulating pipes need covering to reduce the amount of heat loss…

…Waste pipes need covering to prevent them from freezing and to silence the noise caused by the rush of water through them. Ice-water pipes are covered to prevent the water from rising in temperature and to prevent any condensation forming on the pipe…

There are installed on some jobs what is known as an expansion joint. This will allow for the expansion and contraction of the pipe… After a while these joints begin to leak and they must have attention which in some cases is rather expensive. An expansion loop as shown in the sketch, made with elbows, will prove satisfactory. If the threads on the fittings and pipe are good, no leak will appear on this joint.

29. If excessive pressure were to build up in an old boiler that was fitted with a meter, safety valve, and no check valve, then which of the following would most likely occur?

A. An explosion.
B. The meter would break.
C. The boiler would overheat.
D. A leak.

GO ON TO THE NEXT PAGE.

30. According to the passage, hot water flowing through lead pipes would most likely cause:

A. Rust formation.
B. Steam formation.
C. Condensation.
D. Noise.

31. The author's main motivation for writing this passage is to:

A. persuade readers to use appropriate valves and materials.
B. ensure that proper safety measures are in place.
C. provide efficient methods of plumbing.
D. discuss various materials used for pipes, coverings, and storage tanks.

32. The intended audience for this passage is most likely:

A. Inspectors.
B. Engineers.
C. Manufacturers.
D. Residents.

33. One can infer that cold-water pipes need covering in order to:

A. prevent crack formation.
B. reduce the rise in temperatures.
C. silence the noise caused by them.
D. prevent them from freezing.

34. Suppose that a non-dissolvable polymer is applied to the inner lining of pipes, and that the polymer is later found to peel and dislodge. This would most likely cause:

A. Vibrations.
B. Cracking.
C. Snapping.
D. Faster flow.

GO ON TO THE NEXT PAGE.

Passage VII (Questions 35 - 40)

For bookbinding purposes, the sub-committee generally condemns the use of tanning materials belonging to the catechol group, although the leathers produced by the use of these materials are for many purposes excellent, and indeed superior. The class of tanning materials which produce the most suitable leather for this particular purpose belong to the pyrogallol group, of which a well known and important example is sumach.

East Indian or 'Persian' tanned sheep and goat skins, which are suitable for many purposes, and are now used largely for cheap bookbinding purposes, are considered extremely bad. Books bound in these materials have been found to show signs of decay in less than twelve months, and the sub-committee are inclined to believe that no book bound in these leathers, exposed on a shelf to sunlight or gas fumes, can ever be expected to last more than five or six years. Embossing leather under heavy pressure to imitate a grain has a very injurious effect, while the shaving of thick skins greatly reduces the strength of the leather by cutting away the tough fibers of the inner part of the skin. The use of mineral acids in brightening the color of leather, and in the process of dyeing, has a serious effect in lessening its resistance to decay. A good deal yet remains to be learned about the relative permanency of the different dyes.

On analysis free sulphuric acid was found to be present in nearly all bookbinding leather, and it is the opinion of the committee that even a small quantity of this acid materially lessens the durability of the leather.

The publication of the report should tend to fix a standard for bookbinding leather. Hitherto there has been no recognized standard. Bookbinders have selected leather almost entirely by its appearance. It has now been shown that appearance is no test of durability, and the mechanical test of tearing the leather is insufficient. Sound leather should tear with difficulty, and the torn edges should be fringed with long, silky fibers, and any leather which tears very easily, and shows short, curled-up fibers at the torn edges, should be discarded. But though good bookbinding leather will tear with difficulty, and show long fibers where torn, that is in itself not a sufficient test; because it has been shown that the leather that is mechanically the strongest, is not necessarily the most durable and the best able to resist the adverse influences to which books are subject in libraries.

The report shows that bookbinders and librarians are not, as a general rule, qualified to select leather for bookbinding. In the old days, when the manufacture of leather was comparatively simple, a bookbinder might reasonably be expected to know enough of the processes employed to be able to select his leather.

… If librarians will specify that the leather to be employed must be certified to be manufactured according to the recommendations of the Society of Arts Committee, there is no reason why leathers should not be obtained as durable as any ever produced. This would necessitate the examining and testing of batches of leather by experts. At present this can be done more or less privately at various places, such as the Yorkshire College, Leeds, or the Herolds' Institute, Bermondsey. In the near future it is to be hoped that some recognized public body, such as one of the great City Companies interested in leather, may be induced to establish a standard, and to test such leathers as are submitted to them, hall-marking those that come up to the standard. This would enable bookbinders and librarians, in ordering leather, to be sure that it had not been injured in its manufacture. The testing, if done by batches, should not add greatly to the cost of the leather.

GO ON TO THE NEXT PAGE.

35. According to the passage, the following bookbinding processes most likely cause decay EXCEPT:

A. Embossing.
B. Tanning.
C. Brightening.
D. Dyeing.

36. Bookbinders should select leather based on:
  I.   appearance.
  II.   mechanical testing.
  III. durability testing.

A. I only
B. III only
C. I and II only
D. I and III only

37. Which of the following, if true, would most *weaken* the author's claim that librarians are not qualified to select leather?

A. The processing of leather has become more complex.
B. Bookbinding is a relatively simple process.
C. Librarians are involved in the bookbinding process.
D. Leather manufacturers include details of the production process in each book.

38. The passage suggests that a librarian should consider returning a book to its manufacturer if:

A. upon mechanical testing, straight fibers are formed.
B. it is embossed using light pressure.
C. it is made with sheep skin.
D. pages fall out.

39. The author feels confident about the durability of a book if it:

A. tears with difficulty, revealing silky fibers.
B. contains sumach.
C. bears a hall-mark.
D. is acid-free.

40. Suppose that the author used a steel knife that fractured after two years of use. The author would most likely react with:

A. surprise, because steel has high tensile strength.
B. surprise, because a knife should last longer than two years.
C. understanding, because repeated use ruins materials.
D. understanding, because durability depends on strength.

STOP.   IF YOU FINISH BEFORE TIME IS CALLED, CHECK YOUR WORK. YOU MAY GO BACK TO ANY QUESTION IN THIS TEST.

STOP.

Verbal Reasoning Test 3

Time: 60 Minutes
Questions 1 - 40

VERBAL REASONING

DIRECTIONS: There are seven passages in the Verbal Reasoning test. Each passage is followed by five to seven questions. Pace yourself and select the one best answer to each question.

Passage I (Questions 1 - 6)

All routing across the network is done by means of the IP address associated with a packet. Since humans find it difficult to remember addresses like 128.174.5.50, a symbolic name register was set up at the NIC where people would say "I would like my host to be named uiucuxc". Machines connected to the Internet across the nation would connect to the NIC in the middle of the night, check modification dates on the hosts file, and if modified move it to their local machine. With the advent of workstations and micros, changes to the host file would have to be made nightly. It would also be very labor intensive and consume a lot of network bandwidth. RFC-882 and a number of others describe domain name service, a distributed data base system for mapping names into addresses.

We must look a little more closely into what's in a name. First, note that an address specifies a particular connection on a specific network… Second, a machine can have one or more names and one or more network addresses (connections) to different networks. Names point to a something which does useful work (i.e. the machine) and IP addresses point to an interface on that provider. A name is a purely symbolic representation of a list of addresses on the network…

A simplified model of how a name is resolved is that on the user's machine there is a resolver. The resolver knows how to contact across the network a root name server. Root servers are the base of the tree structured data retrieval system. They know who is responsible for

handling first level domains (e.g. 'edu'). What root servers use is an installation parameter. From the root server the resolver finds out who provides 'edu' service. It contacts the 'edu' name server which supplies it with a list of addresses of servers for the subdomains (like 'uiuc').

This action is repeated with the subdomain servers until the final subdomain returns a list of addresses of interfaces on the host in question. The user's machine then has its choice of which of these addresses to use for communication.

A group may apply for its own domain name (like 'uiuc' above). This is done in a manner similar to the IP address allocation. The only requirements are that the requestor have two machines reachable from the Internet, which will act as name servers for that domain. Those servers could also act as servers for subdomains or other servers could be designated as such. Note that the servers need not be located in any particular place, as long as they are reachable for name resolution. (U of I could ask Michigan State to act on its behalf and that would be fine). The biggest problem is that someone must do maintenance on the database. If the machine is not convenient, then maintenance might not be done in a timely fashion. The other thing to note is that once the domain is allocated to an administrative entity, that entity can freely allocate subdomains using whatever manner it sees fit.

1. Suppose a new university applied for its own domain name. Problems would arise if:

A. the university allocated too many machines to act as name servers.
B. the university asked another university to host its name servers
C. the root servers at the university were turned off.
D. too many subdomains were allocated to the domain.

2. What is the correct relationship between names and addresses?

A. If a machine moves to a different network, the addresses will change and the name will change.
B. If a machine moves to a different network, the addresses will change but the name could remain the same.
C. If the machine moves, the address moves with it.
D. Addresses are static.

3. According to the passage, if host files at the NIC did not automatically update their modification dates, then:

A. Machines would check the NIC nightly, but never download updated files.
B. Changes to the host file would have to be made nightly.
C. The NIC would be overwhelmed with machines logging in constantly.
D. Machines would not check the NIC nightly.

4. According to the passage, what is one possible consequence of a mistaken installation parameter?

A. Root servers will point to the wrong resolver.
B. The base of the tree structured data retrieval system will be lost.
C. The resolver will no longer know how to contact across the network.
D. A list of addresses of servers for the subdomains will not be provided.

5. The author would disagree with which of the following statements about network communication?

A. Root servers provide a list of addresses of servers for the subdomains.
B. The same machine can act as a server for both domains and subdomains.
C. A computer can choose which address to use for communication, as provided by the resolver.
D. An allocated domain usually receives one subdomain.

6. Suppose that the author were to teach a course, what is the most likely title for the class?

A. Root Servers 101
B. How to Manage Servers
C. Computers, Resolvers, and Modernization
D. Domains and Subdomains on Campus

GO ON TO THE NEXT PAGE.

Passage II (Questions 7 - 12)

Law, in its original and proper sense, is the expression to an inferior of the will of a superior, which the inferior has it in his power to obey or to resist, but resistance to which entails a penalty more or less severe, in proportion to the moral turpitude, or the injurious consequences of the act of disobedience. In this its strict sense the law can only exist in connection with beings possessed of reason to understand it, of power to obey it, and of free will to determine whether they will obey it or not…

Hence arose in the first instance the term "natural laws," or "laws of nature." …Probably in the minds of those by whom the word was thus applied in the first instance Nature was not the mere abstraction it is now, but an unseen power— Deity or subordinate to Deity— working consciously and with design.

Mr. Darwin, especially in the "Origin of Species," seems continually to betray the existence of this feeling in his own mind. Though he, from time to time, reminds us that by Nature he means nothing but the aggregate of sequences of events, or laws…

Every conscious act is performed under the conviction that the natural forces which that act calls forth will operate in a certain prescribed manner. But this conviction, though it restricts us to the limits of the possible, does not further impede the freedom of our will. To a certain extent we can choose what action we will perform, what forces we will call forth for that purpose, and what direction we will give them. Sometimes we can arrange our forces so that they will continue to act for a considerable time without any intervention from us; in other cases continued interference is necessary. But in all these cases there is no interruption of the law by which the working of these forces is regulated. We have then a limited control over these forces, and yet they are unchangeable in themselves, and in their mode of action.

When, however, we strive to ascend from our own works to those of God, we can no longer regard these forces as absolutely unchangeable. If they are practically so, it is because it is His Will that they should be so. It is this Will then which has its expression in the so-called laws of nature. The term now assumes a sense akin to, though not identical with, its original ethical sense.

It is no longer a rule imposed by a superior on an inferior, but the rule by which the Supreme Being sees fit to order His own Work. While however we admit the possibility of law of this kind being changed, we have no reason to believe that in the universe with which we have to do any such change has ever taken place. But this does not preclude the possibility of Divine interference in the processes either of Creation or of Providence. New forces may from time to time be supplied, new directions may be given to existing forces, without any variation in the laws by which the action of those forces is regulated.

And if we believe that Creation was a progressive act, it is rather probable than otherwise that such interferences should take place. For a long period perhaps the uniformity of the work might lead us to forget the Being who was working… Such interference would not in any way justify the supposition that the designs of the Author of Nature were changed, or that His original plan had proved defective.

GO ON TO THE NEXT PAGE.

7. According to the passage, which of the following is most likely to occur when the three conditions for original law are absent?

A. Only laws of nature will exist.
B. Law in its proper sense will have no existence.
C. Law will remain unchanged.
D. Laws of nature will remain unchanged.

8. What is the best distinction between natural law and Mr. Darwin's concept of law?

A. Original law pertains to civic events. Natural law pertains to observed events.
B. Original law pertains to understandable events. Natural law describes uniform events.
C. Darwin's concept of law pertains to unchangeable events. Natural law describes Divine events.
D. Darwin's concept of law pertains to the sequence of events. Natural law describes Divine events.

9. How would the author account for Divine interference in a world that followed an original plan?

A. Designs of the Author of Nature were part of the plan from the beginning, but that the time for them had not yet come.
B. Designs of the Author of Nature were part of a progressive act, but that the original plan had not changed.
C. Uniformity of the work might lead us to forget the Being who was working, and thus perceive the plan as unchanged.
D. Nature follows an aggregate of sequences of events, which is recognized as Divine interference.

10. The author would most likely agree with which of the following statements about conscious acts?

A. Conscious acts involve deciding which forces to call forth and in what manner, influencing laws of nature.
B. acts ascend from our own works to those of God.
C. Conscious acts operate in a certain prescribed manner that directs human will.
D. Conscious acts operate on predictable natural forces that cannot interrupt natural laws.

11. Suppose that an astronomer discovers that Nature operated like a predictable machine. If true, how would this statement change the meaning of Nature according to the author?

A. The true meaning of the word would be lost.
B. The meaning of the word would not change.
C. The meaning of Nature would expand to include natural events.
D. The meaning of Nature would be complete.

12. The passage suggests that according to the original sense of the word, Nature was the expression of:

A. natural sequences of events.
B. natural phenomenon made by a Creator of order and uniform procedure.
C. natural forces operating in a prescribed manner.
D. natural phenomenon open to influence.

_____

GO ON TO THE NEXT PAGE.

Passage III (Questions 13 - 18)

Taking up these points in order, we shall inquire first into the causes of the agrarian readjustments of the fourteenth century. A generation after the Black Death, the commutation of villain services and the introduction of the leasehold system had made notable progress. The leasing of the demesne has been attributed to the direct influence of the pestilence, which by reducing the serf population made it impossible to secure enough villain labor to cultivate the lord's land. The substitution of money rents in place of the labor services owed by the villains has been explained on the supposition that the serfs who had survived the pestilence took advantage of the opportunity afforded by their reduction in numbers to free themselves from servile labor and thus improve their social status.

The connection between the Black Death and the changes in manorial management which are usually attributed to it could be more convincingly established had not several decades elapsed after the Black Death before these changes became marked. A recent intensive study of the manors of the Bishopric of Winchester during this period confirms the view of those who have protested against assigning to the Black Death the revolutionary importance which is given it by many historians. On these estates the Black Death "produced severe evanescent effects and temporary changes, with a rapid return to the status quo of 1348." The great changes which are usually attributed to the plague of 1348-1350 were under way before 1348, and were not greatly accelerated until 1360, possibly not before 1370…

Levett and Ballard devote especial attention to the effect of the Black Death upon the substitution of money payments for labor services and rents in kind, but their study also brings out the fact that the difficulty in persuading tenants to take up land on the old terms (usually ascribed to the Black Death) began before the pestilence, and continued long after its effects had ceased to exert any influence. Before the Black Death landowners were unable to secure holders for bond land without the use of force. A generation after the Black Death they were still contending with this problem, and it had become more serious than at any previous time…

Holders of land were already deserting, and the tenements of those who died or deserted could frequently be filled only by compulsion. Villains were refusing to perform their services on account of poverty, and they were already securing reductions in their rents and services. The temporary reduction of the population by the Black Death has been advanced as the reason for the ability of the villains of the decade 1350-1360 to enforce their demands; but without the help of any such cause, villains of an earlier period were obtaining concessions from their lords, and after the natural growth of the population had ample time to replace those who had died of the pestilence, the villains were in a stronger position than ever before, if we are to estimate their strength by their success in lightening their economic burdens.

The Black Death at the most did no more than accelerate changes in the tenure of land which were already under way. Villain services were being reduced, and the size of villain holdings increased. The strength of the position of the serfs lay not so much in the absence of competition due to a temporary reduction in their numbers as in their poverty. Tenants could not be held at the accustomed rents and services because it was impossible to make a living from their holdings. The absence of competition for holdings was no temporary thing, due to the high mortality of the years 1348-1350, but was chronic, and was based upon the worthlessness of the land. The vacant tenements of the fourteenth century, the reduction in the area of demesne land planted, the complaints that no profit could be made from tillage, the reduction of rents on account of the poverty of whole villages, all point in the same direction.

GO ON TO THE NEXT PAGE.

13. Which of the following statements, if true, would most *weaken* the study of the manors of the Bishopric of Winchester?

A. Tenants refused to take up land on old terms at the onset of the Black Death, but did so prior to the pestilence.
B. Villains were obtaining concessions from their lords prior to the Black Death.
C. Landowners did not face serious difficulties during the Black Death, but did so prior to the pestilence.
D. The temporary increase in economic burden caused by the Black Death was one reason for the ability of the villains of the decade 1350-1360 to enforce their demands.

14. The passage supports each of the following statements about the Black Death EXCEPT:

A. Serfs desired to improve their social status.
B. Changes in manorial management were gradual.
C. Landowners used less force to secure holders for bond land after the pestilence.
D. Changes in the tenure of land occurred prior to the pestilence.

15. The author would most likely *disagree* with which of the following statements:

A. The pestilence does not explain the events which took place long after its effects were forgotten.
B. The Black Death can explain a condition which arose before its occurrence.
C. One result of the pestilence was to place villains in a stronger position than before.
D. Landowners were already facing serious difficulties before 1348

16. Which of the following does the author consider to be a temporary effect during the mid-fourteenth century?

A. The reduction in the number of serfs.
B. The concessions obtained by villains.
C. The worthlessness of the land.
D. The absence of competition for holdings.

17. Villains were able to secure lower rents by using:

A. poverty as an excuse to refuse services.
B. force against landowners.
C. economic burdens as leverage against serfs.
D. the worthlessness of land as a means to shorten their tenure of the land.

18. One would best characterize the field of occupation of the author as being:

A. political.
B. legal.
C. educational.
D. agrarian.

_____

GO ON TO THE NEXT PAGE.

Passage IV (Questions 19 - 24)

In recent times what we may regard as a new branch of astronomical science is being developed, showing a tendency towards unity of structure throughout the whole domain of the stars. This is what we now call the science of stellar statistics.

The very conception of such a science might almost appall us by its immensity. The widest statistical field in other branches of research is that occupied by sociology.

Every country has its census, in which the individual inhabitants are classified on the largest scale and the combination of these statistics for different countries may be said to include all the interest of the human race within its scope.

Yet this field is necessarily confined to the surface of our planet. In the field of stellar statistics millions of stars are classified as if each taken individually were of no more weight in the scale than a single inhabitant of China in the scale of the sociologist. And yet the most insignificant of these suns may, for aught we know, have planets revolving around it, the interests of whose inhabitants cover as wide a range as ours do upon our own globe.

The outcome of Kapteyn's conclusions is that we are able to describe the universe as a single object, with some characters of an organized whole. A large part of the stars which compose it may be considered as divisible into two groups.

One of these comprises the stars composing the great girdle of the Milky Way. These are distinguished from the others by being bluer in color, generally greater in absolute brilliancy, and affected, there is some reason to believe, with rather slower proper motions.

The other classes are stars with a greater or less shade of yellow in their color, scattered through a spherical space of unknown dimensions, but concentric with the Milky Way. Thus a sphere with a girdle passing around it forms the nearest approach to a conception of the universe which we can reach today. The number of stars in the girdle is much greater than that in the sphere.

Spectroscopic examinations seem to show that all the stars are in motion, and that we cannot say that those in one part of the universe move more rapidly than those in another. This result is of the greatest value for our purpose, because, when we consider only the apparent motions, as ordinarily observed, these are necessarily dependent upon the distance of the star.

We cannot, therefore, infer the actual speed of a star from ordinary observations until we know its distance. But the results of spectroscopic measurements of radial velocity are independent of the distance of the star.

Perhaps the attribute in which the stars show the greatest variety is that of absolute luminosity. The most striking example of this is afforded by the absence of measurable parallaxes in the two bright stars, Canopus and Rigel, showing that these stars, though of the first magnitude, are immeasurably distant.

Rigel has no motion that has certainly been shown by more than a century of observation, and it is not certain that Canopus has either. We may say with certainty that the brightness of each is thousands of times that of the sun ...

On the other hand, there are stars comparatively near us of which the light is not the hundredth part of the sun.

GO ON TO THE NEXT PAGE.

19. What is the main idea of the Canopus and Rigel example?

A. We cannot conclude that because a star is bright, it is near.
B. Parallax cannot measure with reliability the distance of a star.
C. Spectroscopic examination can apply to both near and distant stars.
D. The distances of Canopus and Rigel are immeasurably great.

20. The author most likely views the analogy between stellar statistics and sociology as:

A. appropriate, because both fields classify members by accounting for them individually.
B. imperfect, because stellar statistics cannot account for every planet.
C. apropos, because both fields deal with immense numbers.
D. unbalanced, because stellar statistics does not include all the interest of the human race within its scope.

21. The synthesis of spectroscopic examination, luminosity, and stellar statistics would be most similar to the study of:

A. glowing beetles in a state park.
B. refraction of light through raindrops.
C. luminescent algae in the ocean.
D. solar wind encountering the Earth's atmosphere.

22. According to the passage, the Milky Way is composed primarily of stars with:

A. a shade of yellow, scattered through a spherical space of unknown dimensions, but concentric.
B. greater absolute brilliancy, and rather slower in motion.
C. a shade of blue, composing the great girdle, and faster in motion then stars in the spherical region
D. slower motion and less brilliance than stars in the spherical region.

23. The author would LEAST agree with which of the following observations:

A. The patterns of stellar luminosities support the outcome of Kapteyn's conclusions.
B. Relatively speaking, the sun can be considered a dim or bright star.
C. Observations reveal no motion in Rigel.
D. Apparent motions depend on distance.

24. The author suggests that spectroscopic examination:

A. Could detect different velocities of stars in the girdle and sphere of the Milky Way.
B. Would be applicable to the field of sociology.
C. Could show two stars at different distances as having the same velocities.
D. Could reveal the distances of stars.

GO ON TO THE NEXT PAGE.

Passage V (Questions 25 - 29)

The advent of the Populists as a full-fledged party in the domain of national politics took place at Omaha in July, 1892. Nearly thirteen hundred delegates from all parts of the Union flocked to the convention to take part in the selection of candidates for President and Vice-President and to adopt a platform for the new party. The "Demands" of the Alliances supplied the material from which was constructed a platform characterized by one unsympathetic observer as "that furious and hysterical arraignment of the present times, that incoherent intermingling of Jeremiah and Bellamy."

… It may be suspected, however, that even with Weaver at its head this party, which claimed to control from two to three million votes, and which expected to draw heavily from the discontented ranks of the old-line organizations, was not viewed with absolute equanimity by the campaign managers of Cleveland…

Some little evidence of the perturbation appeared in the equivocal attitude of both the old parties with respect to the silver question. Said the Democratic platform: "We hold to the use of both gold and silver as the standard money of the country, and to the coinage of both gold and silver without discrimination against either metal or charge for mintage."

The rival Republican platform declared that "the American people, from tradition and interest, favor bimetallism, and the Republican party demands the use of both gold and silver as standard money." Each party declared for steps to obtain an international agreement on the question.

The Republicans attempted to throw a sop to the labor vote by favoring restriction of immigration and laws for the protection of employees in dangerous occupations, and to the farmer by pronouncements against trusts, for extended postal service—particularly in rural districts—and for the reclamation and sale of arid lands to settlers.

The Democrats went even further and demanded the return of "nearly one hundred million acres of valuable land" then held by "corporations and syndicates, alien and domestic."

That the tide of agrarianism was gradually flowing westward as the frontier advanced is apparent from the election returns in the States bordering on the upper Mississippi. Iowa and Missouri, where the Alliance had been strong, experienced none of the landslide which swept out the Republicans in States further west. In Minnesota the Populists, with a ticket headed by the veteran Donnelly, ran a poor third in the state election, and the entire Harrison electoral ticket was victorious in spite of the endorsement of four Populist candidates by the Democrats.

In the northwestern part of the State, however, the new party was strong enough to elect a Congressman over candidates of both the old parties. In no Northern State east of the Mississippi were the Populists able to make a strong showing; but in Illinois, the success of John P. Altgeld, the Democratic candidate for governor, was due largely to his advocacy of many of the measures demanded by the People's party, particularly those relating to labor, and to the support which he received from the elements which might have been expected to align themselves with the Populists. On the Pacific coast, despite the musical campaign of Clark, Mrs. Lease, and Weaver, California proved deaf to the People's cause; but in Oregon the party stood second in the lists and in Washington it ran a strong third.

GO ON TO THE NEXT PAGE.

25. According to the passage, the Democrats and Republicans would most likely agree on each of the following EXCEPT:

A. taxes on corporations.
B. immigration.
C. valuable land ownership.
D. the standard money of the country.

26. As implied by the passage, Harrison was most likely running on which ticket?

A. Populist.
B. Republican.
C. Democrat.
D. Independent.

27. What is the main idea of the passage?

A. The 1890s saw the emergence of a new U.S. political party.
B. The Populist party evolved under the leadership of Weaver.
C. The Democrats and Republicans influenced the emergence of the new Populist party.
D. The Populist Party emerged with questionable success.

28. According to the passage, the Populist Party was most successful in which region of the United States?

A. Iowa and Missouri.
B. Illinois.
C. California.
D. Minnesota.

29. The passage is most likely:

A. a transcript from a documentary.
B. an editorial from a local newspaper.
C. an article in a business journal.
D. a report from the Populist Party.

_____

GO ON TO THE NEXT PAGE.

Passage VI (Questions 30 - 35)

The causes which induce the selection of the clerical profession are not often connected with science; and it is, perhaps, a question of considerable doubt whether it is desirable to hold out to its members hopes of advancement from such acquirements. As a source of recreation, nothing can be more fit to occupy the attention of a divine; and our church may boast, in the present as in past times, that the domain of science has been extended by some of its brightest ornaments.

The little encouragement which at all previous periods has been afforded by the English Government to the authors of useful discoveries, or of new and valuable inventions, is justified on the following grounds:
 1. The public, who consume the new commodity or profit by the new invention, are much better judges of its merit than the government can be.
 2. The reward which arises from the sale of the commodity is usually much larger than that which government would be justified in bestowing; and it is exactly proportioned to the consumption, that is, to the want which the public feels for the new article.

Other instances might, if necessary, be adduced, to show that long intervals frequently elapse between the discovery of new principles in science and their practical application: nor ought this at all to surprise us. Those intellectual qualifications, which give birth to new principles or to new methods, are of quite a different order from those which are necessary for their practical application.

At the time of the discovery of the beautiful theorem of Huygens, it required in its author not merely a complete knowledge of the mathematical science of his age, but a genius to enlarge its boundaries by new creations of his own. Such talents are not always united with a quick perception of the details, and of the practical applications of the principles they have developed, nor is it for the interest of mankind that minds of this high order should lavish their powers on subjects unsuited to their grasp.

In mathematical science, more than in all others, it happens that truths which are at one period the most abstract, and apparently the most remote from all useful application, become in the next age the bases of profound physical inquiries, and in the succeeding one, perhaps, by proper simplification and reduction to tables, furnish their ready and daily aid to the artist and the sailor.

It may also happen that at the time of the discovery of such principles, the mechanical arts may be too imperfect to render their application likely to be attended with success. Such was the case with the principle of the hydrostatic paradox; and it was not, I believe, until the expiration of Mr. Bramah's patent, that the press which bears his name received that mechanical perfection in its execution, which has deservedly brought it into such general use.

If, therefore, it is important to the country that abstract principles should be applied to practical use, it is clear that it is also important that encouragement should be held out to the few who are capable of adding to the number of those truths on which such applications are founded. Unless there exist peculiar institutions for the support of such inquirers, or unless the Government directly interfere, the contriver of a thaumatrope may derive profit from his ingenuity, whilst he who unravels the laws of light and vision, on which multitudes of phenomena depend, shall descend unrewarded to the tomb.

Perhaps it may be urged, that sufficient encouragement is already afforded to abstract science in our different universities, by the professorships established at them. It is not however in the power of such institutions to create; they may foster and aid the development of genius; and, when rightly applied, such stations ought to be its fair and honorable rewards. In many instances their emolument is small; and when otherwise, the lectures which are required from the professor are not perhaps in all cases the best mode of employing the energies of those who are capable of inventing.

GO ON TO THE NEXT PAGE.

30. According to the passage, the inventor of a significant theorem must possess which of the following qualifications?

A. quick perception of detail
B. complete knowledge of mathematical science
C. flair for creativity
D. interest in mankind

31. In the context of the passage, the word *ornaments* most nearly means:

A. scientists
B. laity
C. priests
D. members

32. In organizing a society to maximize the number of ideas put to practical use, the author would most likely advise

A. the government to offer tax relief to all inventors in the society.
B. academic institutions to offer professorships to only the inventors of ideas.
C. that a percentage of profits be given to the inventors of ideas on which product are based.
D. that profits be given to the inventors of useful applications that came from abstract ideas.

33. Which of the following statements, if true, would support the author's point about rewarding the originators of ideas?

A. Government profits as much from the invention as does the public.
B. Government is able to judge fully the merit of the invention.
C. Rewards from the sale of the invention are not given to the inventor.
D. Government bestows a greater reward than that which arises from the sale of the commodity to the public.

34. Which of the following statements would the author find most surprising?

A. Universities have a history of creating new ideas.
B. The inventor of the crossbow had complete knowledge of mechanical physics, and the genius of creating a more portable device.
C. Hundreds of years passed between the invention of the wheel, and that of the chariot.
D. Most inventors of ideas are not supported by their governments.

35. A *thaumatrope* most likely refers to:

A. a box that emits a specific pitch of sound when light shines on it.
B. a mechanical violin played by turning a crank.
C. a glass bulb of mercury that rises or falls based on humidity.
D. a card with a picture on each side that is twirled quickly.

GO ON TO THE NEXT PAGE.

Passage VII (Questions 36 - 40)

The difficulty of uniting the farmers of America for any form of co-operative endeavor long ago became proverbial. The business of farming encouraged individualism; comparative isolation bred independence; and restricted means of communication made union physically difficult, even among those who might be disposed to unite. It was not strange, therefore, that the agricultural masses developed a state of mind unfavorable for organization—that they became suspicious of one another, jealous of leadership, unwilling to keep the pledges of union, and unable to sink personal views and prejudices.

It must not be supposed, however, that the farmers themselves have failed to realize the situation, or that no genuinely progressive steps have been taken to remedy it. During the last four decades at least, the strongest men that the rural classes have produced have labored with their fellows, both in season and out of season, for union of effort; and their efforts have been by no means in vain. It is true that some of the attempts at co-operation have been ill-judged, even fantastic. It is true that much of the machinery of organization failed to work and can be found on the social junk-pile, in company with other discarded implements not wholly rural in origin. But it is also true that great progress has been made; that the spirit of co-operation is rapidly emerging as a factor in rural social life; and that the weapons of rural organization have a temper all the better, perhaps, because they were fashioned on the anvil of defeat.

Among all these efforts to unite the farming classes, by far the most characteristic and the most successful is the Grange. The truth of this statement will immediately be questioned by those whose memory recalls the early rush to the Grange, "Granger legislation," and similar phenomena, as well as by those whose impressions have been gleaned from reading the periodicals of the late seventies, when the Grange tide had begun to ebb. Indeed, it seems to be the popular impression that the Grange is not at present a force of consequence, that long ago it became a cripple, if not a corpse. Only a few years ago, an intelligent magazine writer, in discussing the subject of farmers' organizations, made the statement, "The Grange is dead." But the assertion was not true. The popular impression must be revised. The Grange has accomplished more for agriculture than has any other farm organization. Not only is it at the present time active, but it has more real influence than it has ever had before; and it is more nearly a national farmers' organization than any other in existence today.

The Grange is also the oldest of the general organizations for farmers. Though the notion of organizing the farmers was undoubtedly broached early in the history of the country, the germ idea that actually grew into the Grange… should be credited to Mr. O. H. Kelley, a Boston young man who settled on a Minnesota farm in 1849…. In 1866, as agent for the Department of Agriculture, Mr. Kelley made a tour of the South, with the view of gaining a knowledge of the agricultural and mineral resources of that section. On this tour he became impressed with the fact that politicians would never restore peace to the country; that if it came at all, it would have to come through fraternity. As his thought ripened he broached to friends the idea of a "secret society of agriculturists, as an element to restore kindly feelings among the people."

Thus the Grange was born of two needs, one fundamental and the other immediate. The fundamental need of agriculture was that farmers should be better educated for their business; and the immediate need was that of cultivating the spirit of brotherhood between the North and the South. The latter need no longer exists; but the fundamental need still remains and is sufficient excuse for the Grange's existence today.

GO ON TO THE NEXT PAGE.

36. The author's central thesis is that:

A. The business of farming fosters individualism.
B. Farmers develop a state of mind unfavorable for organization.
C. The Grange is the most successful effort to unite the farming class.
D. The Grange was born of two needs.

37. According to the passage, the Grange derives much of its credibility from:

A. the early rush to the Grange.
B. its broad membership.
C. publications.
D. its near national status.

38. According to the passage, the assertion "The Grange is dead" was not true because:

A. it achieved more than any other farm organization.
B. it is still active.
C. it is the oldest general organization for farmers.
D. it reversed the tide of isolation in the farming community.

39. The passage implies each of the following statements about rural organization EXCEPT that:

A. it faced much struggle in its origins.
B. brotherhood now exists between North and South.
C. great progress has been made.
D. organizations previous to the Grange never reached full national status.

40. The example of O. H. Kelly best illustrates the point that:

A. nobody would help agriculturalists except for its own members.
B. farmers called for a secret society of agriculturists.
C. fostering kindly feelings among farmers was the first step towards a solid union.
D. the agricultural masses became suspicious of one another.

STOP.   IF YOU FINISH BEFORE TIME IS CALLED, CHECK YOUR WORK. YOU MAY GO BACK TO ANY QUESTION IN THIS TEST.

STOP.

Verbal Reasoning Test 4

Time: 60 Minutes
Questions 1 - 40

VERBAL REASONING

DIRECTIONS: There are seven passages in the Verbal Reasoning test. Each passage is followed by five to seven questions. Pace yourself and select the one best answer to each question.

Passage I (Questions 1 - 6)

In the first place, society as society does not naturally need a head at all. Its constitution, if left to itself, is not monarchical, but aristocratical. Society, in the sense we are now talking of, is the union of people for amusement and conversation. The making of marriages goes on in it, as it were, incidentally, but its common and main concern is talking and pleasure. There is nothing in this which needs a single supreme head; it is a pursuit in which a single person does not of necessity dominate. By nature it creates an "upper ten thousand"; a certain number of persons and families possessed of equal culture, and equal faculties, and equal spirit, get to be on a level—and that level a high level. By boldness, by cultivation, by "social science" they raise themselves above others; they become the "first families," and all the rest come to be below them. But they tend to be much about a level among one another; no one is recognized by all or by many others as superior to them all…

The faculties which fit a man to be a great ruler are not those of society; some great rulers have been unintelligible like Cromwell, or brusque like Napoleon, or coarse and barbarous like Sir Robert Walpole. The light nothings of the drawing-room and the grave things of office are as different from one another as two human occupations can be. There is no naturalness in uniting the two; the end of it always is, that you put a man at the head of society who very likely is remarkable for social defects, and is not eminent for social merits.

Buckingham Palace is as unlike a club as any place is likely to be. The Court is a separate part, which stands aloof from the rest of the London world, and which has but slender relations with the more amusing part of it. The first two Georges were men ignorant of English, and wholly unfit to guide and lead English society. They both preferred one or two German ladies of bad character to all else in London. George III had no social vices, but he had no social pleasures. He was a family man, and a man of business, and sincerely preferred a leg of mutton and turnips after a good day's work to the best fashion and the most exciting talk. In consequence, society in London, though still in form under the domination of a Court, assumed in fact its natural and oligarchical structure. It, too, has become an "upper ten thousand"; it is no more monarchical in fact than the society of New York.

There may be something in this theory; it may be that the Court of England is not quite as gorgeous as we might wish to see it. But no comparison must ever be made between it and the French Court. The Emperor represents a different idea from the Queen. He is not the head of the State; he IS the State. The theory of his Government is that every one in France is equal, and that the Emperor embodies the principle of equality. The greater you make him, the less, and therefore the more equal, you make all others. He is magnified that others may be dwarfed. The very contrary is the principle of English royalty. As in politics it would lose its principal use if it came forward into the public arena, so in society if it advertised itself it would be pernicious.

1. In order to identify a person to be a great leader of society, the author would most likely look for the following qualities EXCEPT:

A. congeniality.
B. audacity.
C. temperance.
D. cultivation.

2. Suppose the author decided that a head of society were a natural idea for a particular country. Whom would the author advise to lead this country?

A. The head of civil government.
B. The chair of religious affairs.
C. The president of a business.
D. The director of a social club.

3. Which of the following claims is (are) explicitly presented in the passage to justify the supposition that society does not naturally need a head?

    I.   The top level of society naturally overtakes a political leader.
    II.   Organization for communication differs from organization for religious purposes.
    III.   Despite the presence of a Monarchy, society resorts to oligarchic organization.

A. I only
B. III only
C. I and II only
D. I, II and III

4. The author of the passage would support most probably an England where:

A. a King would be the figurehead, and the highest citizens would run the country as political officials.
B. a King would run the entire country.
C. no King would exist, and the highest citizens would run the country as political officials.
D. all citizens would have equal voting power.

5. Which of the following statements, if true, would most *weaken* the author's approval of the French Government?

A. The Emperor promotes himself to higher levels of status and power.
B. The Court of France maintains veto power over the Emperor.
C. A lower class does, in fact, exist in France at this time.
D. Class distinctions broaden as the head of France gains power.

6. Suppose that a citizen of France were asked to compare the Emperor to the Queen of England. The citizen would most likely mention that:

A. The Emperor has the divine right to promote himself more so than does the Queen.
B. The Queen may lead the state, but the Emperor is the state.
C. The Queen is not as powerful as the Emperor.
D. The Emperor is like God, while the Queen is mortal.

GO ON TO THE NEXT PAGE.

Passage II (Questions 7 - 13)

Why do our educated ministers "mourn" when preaching? There are honorable exceptions, but the rule is as stated. We have heard ministers whose educational qualifications were all that could be desired, whose exegeses were faultless, who in their perorations would depart from all standards. They exhume the dead, they picture the beatific splendors of the New Jerusalem, they paint the horrors of hell, they describe deathbed scenes, etc. They do this whether or not it has any connection with the subject in hand. Then it is that the "spirit" comes... I have heard some of our best ministers, and the general statement is true. Our educated ministers are making a serious mistake. This pulpit mannerism is a relic of the days of slavery, and the minister who indulges in it is simply perpetuating a barbarism and is retarding the religious progress of the race. It is true, perhaps, that in most of our congregations large numbers of people love to hear the "tone," but when and how are the people ever to become acquainted with higher religious ideas? How can a minister elevate his congregation when he persistently clings to the practices of thirty years ago?

These ministers seem not to know that nine-tenths of the young, educated, and progressive classes are disgusted with them. This explains the lethargy manifested by the above-minded classes toward the Church. The Church, like all other institutions, must be progressive. The fact that these men are keeping the Church back in the dingy past puts them out of sympathy with it. I recently heard a well-known minister, after howling and ranting and mourning to his heart's content, speak of himself as the "wild presiding elder." He certainly made that impression on several of his audience.

...With many of our unthinking classes it is the "mourn" which they enjoy in the sermons. Instead of carrying home some practical thought and trying to weave it into their lives, they become infatuated with certain tones and give vent to their "feelings" by making the welkin ring. If this is religion, I have been mistaken. If this kind of preaching is an inspiration, it is peculiar to us as a people. If noise and demonstrations are necessary parts of religious worship, then other races are largely wanting in this essential.

The mourning preachers will admit in private that there is no virtue in the mourn, and that they do it simply to "touch up" the old folks. They ought to be ashamed. Such conduct is sinful. They should hate the sins that make them mourn, and drive them from their breast. The religious status of a people is a pretty good index of their civilization. If there are idiosyncrasies in our religious life—in short, if we are not up to the standard—we will be judged accordingly. Though my voice be as one crying in the wilderness, I wish to suggest this religious slogan: "Down with the mourning preacher!"

I doubt if there has ever been an enterprise started by Afro-Americans, no matter how lofty the aim or however honest the intentions, that there were not a few envious souls that stood ready to cry it down. This is to-day the greatest barrier to Afro-American success and the chief reason why we are no further advanced in commercial spheres than we are. In this advanced age of civilization and enlightenment such a state of affairs is sadly to be deplored, for we find that not only among the illiterate class does this exist, but in a greater and more marked degree by those who claim superior intelligence and are looked upon as leaders and shining lights of the race. If one attempts to gain a certain goal, there always stands another ready to pull him back. "You must and shall not get above me" seems to be their fixed motto. Ah! brothers and sisters, you have much yet to learn. If you cannot help another up the hill, you certainly will gain nothing by trying to pull him back. Enviousness is a demon and a monster, and until you learn to live in union and love thy neighbor as thyself, you may never hope to win the respect and esteem of other races.

GO ON TO THE NEXT PAGE.

7. The author would find which of the following most objectionable?

A. A child whining and pretending to cry to persuade others.
B. A policeman yelling at an attacker to cease and desist.
C. An animal growling for no apparent reason.
D. A fog horn signaling ships on a clear day.

8. How would the author complete the following thought? "One of the great mistakes of our religious life is our…"

A. blind trust in clergy.
B. pursuit of progressive culture.
C. mistaking noise for religion.
D. desire to get ahead.

9. The author places the blame for "retarding the religious progress of the race" on the:

A. ministers.
B. church attendees.
C. selfish pursuits.
D. ministers and church attendees.

10. In the passage "the welkin ring" most nearly means:

A. a circle of believers holding hands.
B. a wedding ring.
C. a very loud sound.
D. a bobbin for weaving.

11. The author's argument in the final paragraph compared to the criticism expressed in the earlier portion of the passage is:

A. ironic.
B. satirical.
C. sarcastic.
D. critical.

12. Each of the following statements about ministers is NOT supported by the passage EXCEPT:

A. They are aware of their potentially displeasing styles, and believe some people do not desire them.
B. They are aware of their potentially displeasing styles, but believe some people desire them.
C. They are unaware of their potentially displeasing styles, but believe some people desire them.
D. They are unaware of their potentially displeasing styles, and believe some people do not desire them.

13. The author would most likely compare the experience of the "unthinking classes" attending church to:

A. watching a soap opera.
B. attending a circus.
C. playing a sport.
D. going to sleep.

GO ON TO THE NEXT PAGE.

Passage III (Questions 14 - 19)

How in general are the phenomena of life related to those of the non-living world? How far can we profitably employ the hypothesis that the living body is essentially an automaton or machine, a configuration of material particles, which, like an engine or a piece of clockwork, owes its mode of operation to its physical and chemical construction? It is not open to doubt that the living body is a machine. It is a complex chemical engine that applies the energy of the food-stuffs to the performance of the work of life. But is it something more than a machine? If we may imagine the physico-chemical analysis of the body to be carried through to the very end, may we expect to find at last an unknown something that transcends such analysis and is neither a form of physical energy nor anything given in the physical or chemical configuration of the body? Shall we find anything corresponding to the usual popular conception—which was also along the view of physiologists—that the body is "animated" by a specific "vital principle," or "vital force," … that exists only in the realm of organic nature? If such a principle exists, then the mechanistic hypothesis fails and the fundamental problem of biology becomes a problem sui generis.

I trust that a certain rugged pedagogical virtue in this reply may atone for its lack of elegance. The elephant has a trunk, as the insect has six legs, for the reason that such is the specific nature of the animal; and we may assert with a degree of probability that amounts to practical certainty that this specific nature is the outcome of a definite evolutionary process, the nature and causes of which it is our tremendous task to determine to such extent as we may be able. But this does not yet touch the most essential side of the problem. What is most significant is that the clumsy, short-necked elephant has been endowed—"by nature," as we say—with precisely such an organ, the trunk, as he needs to compensate for his lack of flexibility and agility in other respects. If we are asked why the elephant has a trunk, we must answer because the animal needs it. But does such a reply in itself explain the fact? Evidently not. The question which science

must seek to answer, is how came the elephant to have a trunk; and we do not properly answer it by saying that it has developed in the course of evolution. It has been well said that even the most complete knowledge of the genealogy of plants and animals would give us no more than an ancestral portrait-gallery. We must determine the causes and conditions that have cooperated to produce this particular result if our answer is to constitute a true scientific explanation. And evidently he who adopts the machine-theory as a general interpretation of vital phenomena must make clear to us how the machine was built before we can admit the validity of his theory, even in a single case. Our apparently simple question as to why the animal has a stomach has thus revealed to us the full magnitude of the task with which the mechanist is confronted; and it has brought us to that part of our problem that is concerned with the nature and origin of organic adaptations...

Without attempting adequately to illustrate the nature of organic adaptations, I will direct your attention to what seems to me one of their most striking features regarded from the mechanistic position. This is the fact that adaptations so often run counter to direct or obvious mechanical conditions. Nature is crammed with devices to protect and maintain the organism against the stress of the environment. Some of these are given in the obvious structure of the organism, such as the tendrils by means of which the climbing plant sustains itself against the action of gravity or the winds, the protective shell of the snail, the protective colors and shapes of animals, and the like. Any structural feature that is useful because of its construction is a structural adaptation; and when such adaptations are given the mechanist has for the most part a relatively easy task in his interpretation. He has a far more difficult knot to disentangle in the case of the so-called functional adaptations, where the organism modifies its activities (and often also its structure) in response to changed conditions.

GO ON TO THE NEXT PAGE.

14. The author would explain the long neck of a giraffe most likely by:

A. using the theory of evolution as a model.
B. studying the complete genealogy of giraffes.
C. explaining why the animal needs it.
D. examining the causes and conditions that led to the long neck.

15. The main idea of the mechanistic position is that:

A. adaptations often seem to contradict mechanical conditions.
B. nature is crammed with devices to protect and maintain the organism.
C. adaptations are mechanical responses to the environment.
D. the body has functional adaptations.

16. Each of the following examples represents a structural adaptation that a "mechanist" can readily interpret, EXCEPT:

A. A flatworm cut into two pieces, and each grows into two identical new flatworms.
B. A lizard losing its tail, and growing a new one.
C. A frog using different lungs to breathe in water or on land.
D. An octopus that changes color for camouflage.

17. The attitude of the author towards the concept of "vital force" is best described as:

A. neutral.
B. skeptical.
C. speculative.
D. curious.

18. Based on information in the passage, the author would support each of the following statements EXCEPT:

A. The living body is a machine.
B. Adaptations follow mechanical conditions.
C. Science must look beyond why things exist.
D. Physiologists believe the body is animated.

19. Suppose the lens of an animal's eye, after it is removed, regenerates perfectly but from a different layer of cells than those of the original lens. How would the author respond to this finding?

A. Acknowledge it as support of the mechanistic viewpoint.
B. Be astounded by it, and offer no valid explanation.
C. Suspect it to be erroneous.
D. Accept it as support of evolution.

_____

GO ON TO THE NEXT PAGE.

Passage IV (Questions 20 - 24)

The Protestant Revolution went far to restore the special functions of women to respect. Belief in her individual soul, and in its need of salvation through individual choice, was supplemented by the belief that this choice must be guided by her individual judgment. Celibacy ceased to be a sign of righteousness; and the best men and women married. But beliefs cannot be directly destroyed by revolution; they can only be disturbed and modified. The teachings of Paul, Augustine, Tertullian and St. Jerome were still authoritative, and Calvin and Knox reaffirmed many of them. The family was still subordinate to the Church; and marriage still remained a sacrament, with theological significances, rather than the simple union of a man and woman who loved each other...

But while every new movement in ideas always carries with it other radical ideas, the practical difficulties of mental, social and legal adjustment always prevent the full and harmonious development of all that is involved in any new point of view. In the American colonies the need for new adjustments in religion, government and practical living made it inevitable that any very important change in woman's position should linger. In fact, the student of colonial records finds many traces of ultra conservatism in the treatment of women, though the forces had been liberated which must inevitably open the way for her through the New World of America into a new world of the spirit.

And before the quickening influence of the new life had time to become commonplace, the struggle with England began. The Revolutionary period was a time of intense political education for every one. War and sacrifice glorified the new ideas; and even the children and women could not escape their influence. Why then did not the American Revolution pass on to full freedom and opportunity for women? For the same reason that it did not forever abolish slavery in America. The vested interests involved were so many, and the changes so momentous and difficult...

As conservers of morals and as leaders in higher ideals of life, the advanced women of America came early face to face with two outgrown abuses. One of these was human slavery and the other was intemperance. In attacking these abuses, women had to break with all the traditions that defined their position.

The wealthy and intelligent Englishwoman, Frances Wright, who came to this country in 1818 to attack slavery, found herself doubly opposed because she was a woman speaking in public. Had not St. Paul declared: "It is a shame for women to speak in the church?" Lucretia Mott, born in the Society of Friends in Nantucket, had escaped the full force of this injunction, but even she found, when she attacked slavery in public, that she had invaded a world sacred to men, and she was sternly warned back. Miss Susan B. Anthony also began her public life as a teacher and a temperance reformer. It was only when she found herself helpless, in the presence of the prejudices against her sex, that she turned her attention to freeing women from all purely sex limitation in public life.

In the Civil War, women directly served men; but in the great industrial reorganization which came afterward they served mainly women and children. Here the victories have been won in the press, in the legislative halls, and in courts of law. Working with men, or alone, they have perfected organization, agitated, raised money, printed appeals, and carried cases through the courts, until factories and stores have been made safer, excessive working hours have been cut down, young children have been exempted from labor, many sweat-shops have been closed, and women workers have begun to be organized to care for their own needs.

GO ON TO THE NEXT PAGE.

20. The discussion of the Protestant Revolution shows primarily that:

A. celibacy ceased to be a sign of righteousness.
B. several radical ideas emerged as a consequence.
C. women had to break with the traditions that defined their position.
D. women enjoyed a revival of respect.

21. According to one historian, the French Revolution taught freedom from authority among men and women. If true, the French people would view marriage most likely as a(an):

A. outmoded ceremony.
B. simple union between man and woman.
C. sacrament.
D. legal bond.

22. According to the passage, how were women treated in the American colonies?

A. With full freedom and opportunity.
B. Conservatively, with new opportunities.
C. With few freedoms.
D. In a very restricted fashion, yet with a fresh spirit.

23. The author suggests that each of the following factors motivated women to seek freedom EXCEPT:

A. intemperance.
B. intolerance from men.
C. dissatisfaction with the status of marriage.
D. injustices existing after the Civil War.

24. According to the passage, women did not have full access to opportunities following the American Revolution. How would the author most likely explain this?

A. Many improvements occurred, but the image of women as subordinate to men dominated society during this time.
B. Women did not fight hard enough for effective change, and lost the freedoms they enjoyed during Colonial America.
C. Despite the many interest and momentous changes, only the most imperative needs could receive attention.
D. The abolition of slavery overshadowed the Women's Movement.

_____

GO ON TO THE NEXT PAGE.

Passage V (Questions 25 - 30)

An ancient and famous human institution is in pressing danger. Sir George Campbell has set his face against the time-honored practice of Falling in Love. Parents innumerable, it is true, have set their faces against it already from immemorial antiquity; but then they only attacked the particular instance, without venturing to impugn the institution itself on general principles.

Now this is of course a serious subject, and it ought to be treated seriously and reverently. But, it seems to me, Sir George Campbell's conclusion is exactly the opposite one from the conclusion now being forced upon men of science by a study of the biological and psychological elements in this very complex problem of heredity.

So far from considering love as a 'foolish idea,' opposed to the best interests of the race, I believe most competent physiologists and psychologists, especially those of the modern evolutionary school, would regard it rather as an essentially beneficent and conservative instinct developed and maintained in us by natural causes, for the very purpose of insuring just those precise advantages and improvements which Sir George Campbell thinks he could himself effect by a conscious and deliberate process of selection.

In short, my doctrine is simply the old-fashioned and confiding belief that marriages are made in heaven: with the further corollary that heaven manages them, one time with another, a great deal better than Sir George Campbell.

Falling in Love, as modern biology teaches us to believe, is nothing more than the latest, highest, and most involved exemplification, in the human race, of that almost universal selective process which Mr. Darwin has enabled us to recognize throughout the whole long series of the animal kingdom. We do fall in love, taking us in the lump, with the young, the beautiful, the strong, and the healthy; we do not fall in love, taking us in the lump, with the aged, the ugly, the feeble, and the sickly. The prohibition of the Church is scarcely needed to prevent a man from marrying his grandmother. Moralists have always borne a special grudge to pretty faces; but, as Mr. Herbert Spencer admirably put it (long before the appearance of Darwin's selective theory), 'the saying that beauty is but skin-deep is itself but a skin-deep saying.'

What we all fall in love with, then, as a race, is in most cases efficiency and ability. What we each fall in love with individually is, I believe, our moral, mental, and physical complement. Not our like, not our counterpart; quite the contrary; within healthy limits, our unlike and our opposite.

Brothers and sisters have more in common, mentally and physically, than any other members of the same race can possibly have with one another. But nobody falls in love with his sister. Of course we do not definitely seek out and discover such qualities; instinct works far more intuitively than that; but we find at last, by subsequent observation, how true and how trustworthy were its immediate indications.

We are not all created in pairs, like the Exchequer tallies, exactly intended to fit into one another's minor idiosyncrasies. Men and women as a rule very sensibly fall in love with one another in the particular places and the particular societies they happen to be cast among.

A man at Ashby-de-la-Zouch does not hunt the world over to find his pre-established harmony at Paray-le-Monial or at Denver, Colorado. But among the women he actually meets, a vast number are purely indifferent to him; only one or two, here and there, strike him in the light of possible wives, and only one in the last resort (outside Salt Lake City) approves herself to his inmost nature as the actual wife of his final selection.

GO ON TO THE NEXT PAGE.

25. The passage suggests that the most favorable portrayal Sir George Campbell gave of Falling in Love was to interpret it as:

A. the best interest of the race.
B. a universal selective process.
C. skin deep.
D. psychological folly.

26. Suppose Sir George Campbell announced that beauty is one of the very best guides we can possibly have to the desirability of any man or any woman as a partner in marriage. How would this information affect the author's claims about modern biology?

A. It would support the claim that modern biology causes people to seek their moral, mental, and physical complement.
B. It would weaken the claim that modern biology causes people to fall in love in particular places and particular societies they happen to be cast among.
C. It would support the claim that modern biology follows a ubiquitous selection process.
D. It would weaken the claim that modern biology protects love as an essentially beneficent and conservative instinct developed and maintained in us by natural causes.

27. The passage suggests that, before the time of physiologists and psychologists of the modern evolutionary school, experts regarded the act of Falling in Love as:

A. a conservative instinct.
B. foolish and not useful.
C. not clearly beneficial.
D. a controllable, deliberate process of selection.

28. The passage as a whole suggests that in order to find true happiness, people must:

A. fall in love with their counterpart.
B. seek out their true complement.
C. meet someone of opposite constitution who appeals to their innermost nature.
D. fall in love with someone of the same class in society.

29. The tone of the author towards Sir George Campbell can be best described as being:

A. satirical and instructive.
B. smug, yet polite.
C. disapproving and ironic.
D. blithe, yet critical.

30. According to the passage, men and women fall in love:

A. in the class they find themselves in.
B. with someone who pays much attention to the other person.
C. when biology determines it to happen.
D. unexpectedly.

GO ON TO THE NEXT PAGE.

Passage VI (Questions 31 - 35)

The eclipse occurred later than calculation warrants. Now this would have happened from either of two causes, either an acceleration of the moon in her orbit, or a retardation of the earth in her diurnal rotation—a shortening of the month or a lengthening of the day, or both.

The total discrepancy being, say, two hours, an acceleration of six seconds-per-century per century will in thirty-six centuries amount to one hour; and this, according to the corrected Laplacian theory, is what has occurred. But to account for the other hour some other cause must be sought, and at present it is considered most probably due to a steady retardation of the earth's rotation—a slow, very slow, lengthening of the day.

The statement that a solar eclipse thirty-six centuries ago was an hour late, means that a place on the earth's surface came into the shadow one hour behind time— that is, had lagged one twenty-fourth part of a revolution .... The loss per revolution is exceedingly small, but it accumulates, and at any era the total loss is the sum of all the losses preceding it.

Winds and ocean currents have no such effect because they are all accompanied by a precisely equal counter-current somewhere else, and no internal rearrangement of fluid can affect the motion of a mass as a whole; but the tides are a different case, being produced, not by internal inequalities of temperature, but by a straightforward pull from an external body.
In so far as the tidal wave is allowed to oscillate freely, it will swing with barely any maintaining force, giving back at one quarter-swing what it has received at the previous quarter; but in so far as it encounters friction, which it does in all channels where there is an actual ebb and flow of the water, it has to receive more than it gives back... The energy of the tides is, in fact, continually being dissipated by friction, and all the energy so dissipated is taken from the rotation of the earth.

The system is disturbed by the tide-generating force of the sun. It is a small effect, but it is cumulative; and gradually, by much slower degrees than anything we have yet contemplated, we are presented with a picture of the month getting gradually shorter than the day.

Mars' principal moon circulates around it at an absurd pace, completing a revolution in 7 1/2 hours, and it is now only 4,000 miles from his surface. The planet rotates in twenty-four hours as we do; but its tides are following its moon more quickly than it rotates after them; they are therefore tending to increase its rate of spin, and to retard the revolution of the moon.

Mars is therefore slowly but surely pulling its moon down on to itself ... The day shorter than the month forces a moon further away; the month shorter than the day tends to draw a satellite nearer.

Tides are of course produced in the sun by the action of the planets, for the sun rotates in twenty-five days or thereabouts, while the planets revolve in much longer periods than that.

The principal tide-generating bodies will be Venus and Jupiter; the greater nearness of one rather more than compensating for the greater mass of the other.
We have been speaking of millions of years somewhat familiarly; but what, after all, is a million years that we should not speak familiarly of it? It is longer than our lifetime, it is true. No less are we compelled to recognize the existence of incalculable eons of time, and yet to perceive that these are but as drops in the ocean of eternity.

GO ON TO THE NEXT PAGE.

31. Which of the following statements weaken the argument of the author?

    I.   If the balance of energy of a tidal wave were to become disrupted, the tides would cease.

    II.   If tidal energy were utilized by engineers, the machines driven would be driven at the expense of the earth's rotation.

    III.   Hot air currents in Earth's atmosphere cause the rotation of Earth to slow ever so slightly.

A. I only
B. III only
C. I and III only
D. I, II and III

32. Suppose that in 7,200 years, a solar eclipse will occur on Earth. Compared to today, a place on the Earth's surface will come into the shadow:

A. 4 hours late.
B. 2 hours early.
C. 2 hours late.
D. 3 hours early.

33. A supporter of the theory about Mars and its moon would most likely believe that the Earth will:

A. collide eventually with the moon.
B. draw closer but never collide with the moon due to the pull of neighboring planets.
C. be pulled further apart from the moon.
D. increase its rate of spin, and retard the revolution of the moon.

34. This passage would most likely appear in what format?

A. newspaper
B. letter from the editor in a journal
C. academic lecture
D. textbook

35. Each of the following statements is supported by an explanation or example in the passage EXCEPT:

A. Mankind is capable of recognizing eternity.
B. The length of day of Mars' moon is increasing.
C. A distant, yet massive planet will have the same effect on tides as a smaller, closer planet.
D. If a solar eclipse thirty-six centuries ago was an hour early, then a place on the earth's surface came into the shadow one hour ahead of time.

_____

GO ON TO THE NEXT PAGE.

Passage VII (Questions 36 - 40)

The right of secession is not claimed as a revolutionary right, or even as a conventional right…

Secession is simply the repeal by the State of the act of accession to the Union; and as that act was a free, voluntary act of the State, she must always be free to repeal it. The Union is a copartnership; a State in the Union is simply a member of the firm, and has the right to withdraw when it judges it for its interest to do so. There is no power in a firm to compel a copartner to remain a member any longer than he pleases…

The population is fixed to the domain and goes with it; the domain is attached to the State, and secedes in the secession of the State. Secession, then, carries the entire State government, people, and domain out of the Union, and restores ipso facto the State to its original position of a sovereign State, foreign to the United States. Being an independent sovereign State, she may enter into a new confederacy, form a new copartnership, or merge herself in some other foreign state, as she judges proper or finds opportunity…

This is the secession argument, which rests on no assumption of revolutionary principles or abstract rights of man, and on no allegation of real or imaginary wrongs received from the Union, but simply on the original and inherent rights of the several States as independent sovereign States…

Until erected into States and admitted into the Union, this territory, with its population, though subject to the United States, makes no part of the political or sovereign territory and people of the United States. It is under the Union, not in it, as is indicated by the phrase admitting into the Union—

But this one sovereign people that exists only as organized into States, does not necessarily include the whole population or territory included within the jurisdiction of the United States. It is restricted to the people and territory or domain organized into States in the Union, as in ancient Rome the ruling people were restricted to the tenants of the sacred territory, which had been surveyed, and its boundaries marked by the god Terminus, and which by no means included all the territory held by the city, and of which she was both the private proprietor and the public sovereign. The city had vast possessions acquired by confiscation, by purchase, by treaty, or by conquest, and in reference to which her celebrated agrarian laws were enacted, and which have their counterpart in our homestead and kindred laws. In this class of territory, of which the city was the private owner, was the territory of all the Roman provinces, which was held to be only leased to its occupants, who were often dispossessed, and their lands given as recompense by the consul or imperator to his disbanded legionaries. The provincials were subjects of Rome, but formed no part of the Roman people, and had no share in the political power of the state, until at a late period the privileges of Roman citizens were extended to them, and the Roman people became coextensive with the Roman Empire…

The Territory gives up no sovereign powers by coming into the Union, for before it came into the Union it had no sovereignty, no political rights at all. All the rights and powers it holds are held by the simple fact that it has become a State in the Union. This is as true of the original States as of the new States; for it has been shown… that the original British sovereignty under which the colonies were organized and existed passed, on the fact of independence, to the States United, and not to the States severally.

GO ON TO THE NEXT PAGE.

36. Which statement, if true, would most *weaken* the argument of the secessionists?

A. Sovereignty vests not in the States severally, but in the States united, or that the Union is sovereign, and not the States individually.
B. The Union is not a firm, a copartnership, nor an artificial or conventional union.
C. Sovereignty vests in the States severally, and the Union is a partnership.
D. The Union, like a firm, has the power to compel its members to remain.

37. The author uses the example of Roman jurisdiction to make which point about territories in the United States?

A. A territory of the United States is automatically a part of the nation's political population.
B. A territory can be subject to the United States, but makes no part of the political population until admitted into the Union.
C. A territory cannot be subject to the United States without redefining its boundaries.
D. A territory of the United States becomes admitted into the Union when privileges of US citizens are extended to it.

38. The author would view the citizens of states who revolt for secession as:

A. revolutionists.
B. sovereign citizens.
C. traitors.
D. patriots.

39. Referring to the thirteen states of the original United States as mentioned in the final paragraph, suppose nine states ratify the constitution and four do not. How would the author view the status of the states that refuse to sign?

A. The four states step beyond their rights and competency.
B. The four become independent sovereign States.
C. The four states default to territories under the Union.
D. The four states become privately held territories.

40. The author would most likely support all of the following statements EXCEPT:

A. The Union does not have jurisdiction over the whole population who live in the United States.
B. The State relinquishes its rights when it enters the Union.
C. The Union is not formed by the surrender to it by the several States of their respective individual sovereignty.
D. Provincials are subjects of a nation and do not necessarily comprise its people.

STOP.   IF YOU FINISH BEFORE TIME IS CALLED, CHECK YOUR WORK. YOU MAY GO BACK TO ANY QUESTION IN THIS TEST.

STOP.

Verbal Reasoning Test 5

Time: 60 Minutes
Questions 1 - 40

VERBAL REASONING

DIRECTIONS: There are seven passages in the Verbal Reasoning test. Each passage is followed by five to seven questions. Pace yourself and select the one best answer to each question.

Passage I (Questions 1 - 5)

In Plato's Laws it is however different; we shall mention hereafter what we think would be best in these particulars. He has also neglected in that treatise to point out how the governors are to be distinguished from the governed; for he says, that as of one sort of wool the warp ought to be made, and of another the wool, so ought some to govern, and others to be governed. But since he admits, that all their property may be increased fivefold, why should he not allow the same increase to the country? he ought also to consider whether his allotment of the houses will be useful to the community, for he appoints two houses to each person, separate from each other; but it is inconvenient for a person to inhabit two houses.

Now he is desirous to have his whole plan of government neither a democracy nor an oligarchy, but something between both, which he calls a polity, for it is to be composed of men-at-arms. If Plato intended to frame a state in which more than in any other everything should be common, he has certainly given it a right name; but if he intended it to be the next in perfection to that which he had already framed, it is not so; for perhaps some persons will give the preference to the Lacedaemonian form of government, or some other which may more completely have attained to the aristocratic form.

Some persons say, that the most perfect government should be composed of all others blended together, for which reason they commend that of Lacedaemon; for

they say, that this is composed of an oligarchy, a monarchy, and a democracy, their kings representing the monarchical part, the senate the oligarchical; and, that in the ephori may be found the democratical, as these are taken from the people. But some say, that in the ephori is absolute power, and that it is their common meal and daily course of life, in which the democratical form is represented.

It is also said in this treatise of Laws, that the best form of government must, be one composed of a democracy and a tyranny; though such a mixture no one else would ever allow to be any government at all, or if it is, the worst possible; those propose what is much better who blend many governments together; for the most perfect is that which is formed of many parts.

But now in this government of Plato's there are no traces of a monarchy, only of an oligarchy and democracy; though he seems to choose that it should rather incline to an oligarchy, as is evident from the appointment of the magistrates; for to choose them by lot is common to both; but that a man of fortune must necessarily be a member of the assembly, or to elect the magistrates, or take part in the management of public affairs, while others are passed over, makes the state incline to an oligarchy; as does the endeavoring that the greater part of the rich may be in office, and that the rank of their appointments may correspond with their fortunes.

The same principle prevails also in the choice of their senate; the manner of electing which is favorable

GO ON TO THE NEXT PAGE.

also to an oligarchy; for all are obliged to vote for those who are senators of the first class, afterwards they vote for the same number out of the second, and then out of the third; but this compulsion to vote at the election of senators does not extend to the third and fourth classes and the first and second class only are obliged to vote for the fourth. By this means he says he shall necessarily have an equal number of each rank, but he is mistaken—for the majority will always consist of those of the first rank, and the most considerable people; and for this reason, that many of the commonalty not being obliged to it, will not attend the elections.

1. Which statement about Plato's concept of government is incorrect?

A. The polity is less perfect than Plato's previous constructs.
B. Governance should not include tyranny.
C. Monarchies are not of serious consideration.
D. Governance tends towards oligarchies.

2. The political state described in the final paragraph:

A. mimics the Lacedaemonian form of government.
B. reduces the power of the senate.
C. will not consist of a democracy and a monarchy.
D. gives the majority of control to the magistrates.

3. All of the following forms of government were described in the passage EXCEPT:

A. a combination of democracy, oligarchy, and monarchy.
B. a combination of democracy and oligarchy, without any monarchy.
C. a combination of democracy and monarchy, without any oligarchy.
D. a semi-democracy and semi-oligarchy.

4. According to the author, what do ephori and polity have in common?

A. some essence or form of democracy.
B. guardianship by men-at-arms.
C. approval from the senate.
D. absolute power.

5. Which of the following circumstances favors democracy over oligarchy?

A. All are obliged to vote for senators of all four classes.
B. A king is elected by popular vote by all people.
C. Commoners vote for their own representatives in a Lacedaemonian form of government.
D. Senators from the third and fourth classes vote for representatives from the commonality.

GO ON TO THE NEXT PAGE.

Passage II (Questions 6 - 11)

The true explanation is, I think, something like this. One considerable writer gets a sort of start because what he writes is somewhat more—only a little more very often, as I believe—congenial to the minds around him than any other sort. This writer is very often not the one whom posterity remembers—not the one who carries the style of the age farthest towards its ideal type, and gives it its charm and its perfection. It was not Addison who began the essay-writing of Queen Anne's time, but Steele; it was the vigorous forward man who struck out the rough notion, though it was the wise and meditative man who improved upon it and elaborated it, and whom posterity reads…

But definitely aimed mimicry like this is always rare; original men who like their own thoughts do not willingly clothe them in words they feel they borrow. No man, indeed, can think to much purpose when he is studying to write a style not his own…

Most men catch the words that are in the air, and the rhythm which comes to them they do not know from whence; an unconscious imitation determines their words, and makes them say what of themselves they would never have thought of saying…

A writer does not begin to write in the traditional rhythm of an age unless he feels, or fancies he feels, a sort of aptitude for writing it, any more than a writer tries to write in a journal in which the style is uncongenial or impossible to him. Indeed if he mistakes he is soon weeded out; the editor rejects, the age will not read his compositions. How painfully this traditional style cramps great writers whom it happens not to suit, is curiously seen in Wordsworth, who was bold enough to break through it, and, at the risk of contemporary neglect, to frame a style of his own. But he did so knowingly, and he did so with an effort…

A strict, I was going to say a Puritan, genius will act thus, but most men of genius are susceptible and versatile, and fall into the style of their age…

What writers are expected to write, they write; or else they do not write at all; but, like the writer of these lines, stop discouraged, live disheartened, and die leaving fragments which their friends treasure, but which a rushing world never heeds. The Nonconformist writers are neglected, the Conformist writers are encouraged, until perhaps on a sudden the fashion shifts. And as with the writers, so in a less degree with readers. Many men—most men—get to like or think they like that which is ever before them, and which those around them like, and which received opinion says they ought to like; or if their minds are too marked and oddly made to get into the mold, they give up reading altogether, or read old books and foreign books, formed under another code and appealing to a different taste.

6. According to the passage, how will the average genius writer approach the task of writing about sailing for two separate newspapers?

A. The writer will write with a style that catches the tone of one newspaper, and then change the style of the article to catch the tone of the other newspaper.

B. The writer will write with a style that departs from the tone of one newspaper, and then change the style of the article to catch the tone of the other newspaper.

C. The writer will write two different articles using the same tone in each piece, and submit them to the newspapers.

D. The writer will submit the same article to both newspapers. The style of the article will differ from the style of either newspaper in order to create a new style.

GO ON TO THE NEXT PAGE.

7. The passage implies that a new writer emerges from competing writers when:

A. The new writer mimics the style of a currently famous author.
B. The new writer unconsciously imitates the style of a currently famous author.
C. The new writer is bold enough to break through and create a style of his own.
D. The new writer's style imprints itself upon the memories of people more so than that of other writers.

8. According to the passage, under what circumstances would an original Nonconformist writer become an original Conformist writer?

A. When the Nonconformist writer, sensing a shift in the popular style, changes his style to meet that shift.
B. When the popular style happens to shift to a style that matches that of the Nonconformist.
C. When the popular style happens to shift away from the Conformist's style.
D. When the Conformist writer, sensing a shift in the popular style, fails to change his style to meet that shift.

9. The tone of the author is best described as:

A. instructive.
B. insensitive.
C. sympathetic.
D. persuasive.

10. Suppose it was discovered that national character emerges in a similar fashion to that of popular literary style. How would the author describe the emergence of America's national character?

A. A chance predominance of character arising from colonial life, and the society unconsciously imitating it.
B. A predominance of character arising from a political leader in colonial life, and the society unconsciously imitating it.
C. A chance predominance of character arising from colonial life, and the political leader of the society imitating it.
D. A predominance of character arising from a political leader in colonial life, and the future elected leaders imitating it.

11. How would the author best describe human instinct?

A. The human mind tends to mimic what is around it.
B. The human spirit has an innate tendency to break from popular style.
C. The human mind has an inherent desire to mimic a mold, whether that mold is imposed or not.
D. The human spirit will not peruse something that is not popular.

_____

GO ON TO THE NEXT PAGE.

Passage III (Questions 12 - 16)

In the monastic confines of the Massachusetts Institute of Technology, people had the freedom to live out this dream—the hacker dream. No one dared suggest that the dream might spread. Instead, people set about building, right there at MIT, a hacker Xanadu the likes of which might never be duplicated…

So Wagner began working on a computer program that would emulate the behavior of a calculator. The idea was outrageous. To some, it was a misappropriation of valuable machine time. According to the standard thinking on computers, their time was too precious that one should only attempt things which took maximum advantage of the computer, things that otherwise would take roomfuls of mathematicians days of mindless calculating. Hackers felt otherwise: anything that seemed interesting or fun was fodder for computing— and using interactive computers, with no one looking over your shoulder and demanding clearance for your specific project, you could act on that belief.

After two or three months of tangling with intricacies of floating-point arithmetic (necessary to allow the program to know where to place the decimal point) on a machine that had no simple method to perform elementary multiplication, Wagner had written three thousand lines of code that did the job. He had made a ridiculously expensive computer perform the function of a calculator that cost a thousand times less. To honor this irony, he called the program Expensive Desk Calculator, and proudly did the homework for his class on it.

Kotok, though, recognized that because of the huge amounts of numbers that would have to be crunched in a chess program, part of the program would have to be done in FORTRAN, and part in assembly. They hacked it part by part, with "move generators," basic data structures, and all kinds of innovative algorithms for strategy. After feeding the machine the rules for moving each piece, they gave it some parameters by which to evaluate its position, consider various moves, and make the move which would advance it to the most advantageous situation. Kotok kept at it for years, the program growing as MIT kept upgrading its IBM computers, and one memorable night a few hackers gathered to see the program make some of its first moves in a real game. Its opener was quite respectable, but after eight or so exchanges there was real trouble, with the computer about to be checkmated.

Everybody wondered how the computer would react. It took a while (everyone knew that during those pauses the computer was actually "thinking," if your idea of thinking included mechanically considering various moves, evaluating them, rejecting most, and using a predefined set of parameters to ultimately make a choice). Finally, the computer moved a pawn two squares forward—illegally jumping over another piece. A bug! But a clever one—it got the computer out of check. Maybe the program was figuring out some new algorithm with which to conquer chess.

But they would not be the only beneficiaries. Everyone could gain something by the use of thinking computers in an intellectually automated world. And wouldn't everyone benefit even more by approaching the world with the same inquisitive intensity, skepticism toward bureaucracy, openness to creativity, unselfishness in sharing accomplishments, urge to make improvements, and desire to build as those who followed the Hacker Ethic? By accepting others on the same unprejudiced basis by which computers accepted anyone who entered code into a Flexowriter? Wouldn't we benefit if we learned from computers the means of creating a perfect system? If everyone could interact with computers with the same innocent, productive, creative impulse that hackers did, the Hacker Ethic might spread through society like a benevolent ripple…

12. Suppose that professors were making public proclamations that computers would never be able to beat a human being in chess. How would hackers respond to this claim?

A. They would reject the claim and attempt to build the best chess program possible.
B. They would consider a chess program a misappropriation of valuable machine time.
C. They would remain quiet to maintain their positions in academia.
D. They would build a bug to beat a human player.

13. Which of the following, if true, would most likely change the author's attitude towards the Hacker Ethic?

A. Programs built by hackers benefit computers.
B. Hackers write programs in FORTRAN.
C. Hackers create programs that harm users of computers.
D. Hackers create bugs inadvertently which have unpredictable consequences.

14. Suppose a hacker built a program for a Mars rover to drive around obstacles on the ground. How would the program work?

A. The rover would stop in front of the obstacle, evaluate the best path, reject other paths, and use parameters to choose the ultimate path.
B. The rover would stop in front of the obstacle, evaluate paths around it, reject the longest path, and use parameters to choose the ultimate path.
C. The rover would stop in front of the obstacle, evaluate the best path, reject the longest path, and use parameters to choose the ultimate path.
D. The rover would stop in front of the obstacle, evaluate paths around it, reject most, and use parameters to choose the ultimate path.

15. The following statements are supported by the author EXCEPT:

A. Kotok spent years building the chess program.
B. Without floating-point arithmetic, the program will not know where to place the decimal point.
C. A bug caused one pawn to jump over another pawn.
D. Wagner used assembly to build a computer program.

16. The author is most likely a:

A. hacker.
B. chess player.
C. mathematician.
D. computer scientist.

_____

GO ON TO THE NEXT PAGE.

Passage IV (Questions 17 - 23)

Cut off a lizard's tail, and straightway a new tail grows in its place with surprising promptitude. Cut off a lobster's claw, and in a very few weeks that lobster is walking about airily on his native rocks, with two claws as usual.

True, in these cases the tail and the claw don't bud out and turn into a new lizard or a new lobster. But that is a penalty the higher organisms have to pay for their extreme complexity. They have lost that plasticity, that freedom of growth, which characterizes the simpler and more primitive forms of life; in their case the power of producing fresh organisms entire from a single fragment, once diffused equally over the whole body, is now confined to certain specialized cells ... Yet, even among animals, at a low stage of development, this original power of reproducing the whole from a single part remains inherent in the organism; for you may chop up a fresh-water hydra into a hundred little bits, and every bit will be capable of growing afresh into a complete hydra.

Now, desert plants would naturally retain this primitive tendency in a very high degree; for they are specially organized to resist drought—-being the survivors of generations of drought-proof ancestors— and, like the camel, they have often to struggle on through long periods of time without a drop of water.

That is why the prickly pear is so common in all countries where the climate suits it, and where it has once managed to gain a foothold. The more you cut it down, the thicker it springs ... Man, however, with his usual ingenuity, has managed to best the plant, on this its own ground, and turn it into a useful fodder for his beasts of burden.

The prickly pear is planted abundantly on bare rocks in Algeria, where nothing else would grow, and is cut down when adult, divested of its thorns by a rough process of hacking, and used as food for camels and cattle. It thus provides fresh moist fodder in the African summer when the grass is dried up and all other pasture crops have failed entirely.

Both the prickly-pear cactus and the American agave have spread themselves in an apparently wild condition over all the rocky coasts both of Southern Europe and of Northern Africa. But for the origin, and therefore for the evolutionary history, of either plant, we must look away from the shore of the inland sea to the arid expanse of the Mexican desert. It was there, among the sweltering rocks of the Tierras Calientes, that these ungainly cactuses first learned to clothe themselves in prickly mail, to store in their loose tissues an abundant supply of sticky moisture, and to set at defiance the persistent attacks of all external enemies ... As far as their leaf-like stems go, the main object in life of the cactuses is—not to get eaten.

That belt of dry beach that stretches between high-water mark and the zone of vegetable mold, is to all intents and purpose a miniature desert. True, it is watered by rain from time to time; but the drops sink in so fast that in half an hour, as we know, the entire strip is as dry as Sahara again ... One such weed, the common salicornia, which grows in sandy bottoms or hollows of the beach, has a jointed stem, branched and succulent ... and entirely without leaves or their equivalents in any way ... The glasswort has leaves, it is true, but they are thick and fleshy, continuous with the stem, and each one terminating in a sharp, needle-like spine, which effectually protects the weed against all browsing aggressors.

It is a marked characteristic of the cactus tribe to be very tenacious of life, and when hacked to pieces, to spring afresh in full vigor from every scrap or fragment ... Surprising as this peculiarity seems at first sight, it is only a special desert modification of a faculty possessed in a less degree by almost all plants and by many animals ... one may say that every fragment of every organism has in it the power to rebuild in its entirety another organism like the one of which it once formed a component element.

GO ON TO THE NEXT PAGE.

17. The passage as a whole suggests that in order for a plant to grow without soil, it must:

A. possess spines and thick leaves, grow on rocks, and be exposed to rain from time to time.
B. grow on rocks, possess a prickly covering, and survive without a drop of water.
C. grow new plants after being scattered, survive without a drop of water, and possess needles.
D. multiply rapidly, retain moisture, and be exposed to rain from time to time.

18. The claim that higher organisms pay a penalty for their extreme complexity is based mainly on the:

A. examinations of sea life and desert life.
B. studies of lizards and lobsters.
C. observations of desert plants and animals.
D. analyses of lobsters, lizards, and prickly pears.

19. The salicornia is cited in the passage as support for the inference that:

A. many shore weeds of the intermediate sand-belt mimic to a surprising degree the chief external features of the cactuses.
B. many shore weeds have a tendency to produce rounded stems and leaves.
C. many shore weeds below the zone of vegetable mold are similar to the prickly pear.
D. many shore weeds above the high-water mark have in them the ability to rebuild in its entirety another organism

20. Which of the following statements, if true, would most *weaken* the conclusions of the author?

A. True vegetable hydras, when you cut down one, ten spring in its place.
B. Every separate morsel of thick and succulent stems of desert plants has the power of growing into a separate cactus.
C. The prickly pear is designed for its fruit to be devoured by birds and animals.
D. All plants in regions starved of rain survive by accessing underground water.

21. As suggested by the passage, which of the following features are characteristic of most plants and animals?

    I.   Defense mechanisms to not get eaten.
    II.   The tendency to preserve water.
    III. The power to regenerate in its entirety another organism.

A. I only
B. II only
C. I and III only
D. II and III only

22. The tone of the author is best described as:

A. ironic.
B. curious.
C. instructive.
D. fascinated.

23. In the context of the passage, the word *best* means:

A. hybridize.
B. defeat.
C. isolate.
D. remove.

GO ON TO THE NEXT PAGE.

Passage V (Questions 24 - 28)

…in the first place, we see that all cities are made up of families: and again, of the multitude of these some must be rich, some poor, and others in the middle station; and that, both of the rich and poor, some will be used to arms, others not. We see also, that some of the common people are husbandmen, others attend the market, and others are artificers. There is also a difference between the nobles in their wealth…

It is evident then, that there must be many forms of government, differing from each other in their particular constitution: for the parts of which they are composed each differ from the other. For government is the ordering of the magistracies of the state; and these the community share between themselves, either as they can attain them by force, or according to some common equality which there is amongst them, as poverty, wealth, or something which they both partake of…

…And these seem chiefly to be two, as they say, of the winds: namely, the north and the south; and all the others are declinations from these.

And thus in politics, there is the government of the many and the government of the few; or a democracy and an oligarchy: for an aristocracy may be considered as a species of oligarchy, as being also a government of the few; and what we call a free state may be considered as a democracy: as in the winds they consider the west as part of the north, and the east as part of the south.

And thus it is in music, according to some, who say there are only two species of it, the Doric and the Phrygian, and all other species of composition they call after one of these names; and many people are accustomed to consider the nature of government in the same light; but it is both more convenient and more correspondent to truth to distinguish governments as I have done, into two species: one, of those which are established upon proper principles of which there may be one or two sorts.

The other… includes all the different excesses of these; so that we may compare the best form of government to the most harmonious piece of music; the oligarchic and despotic to the more violent tunes; and the democratic to the soft and gentle airs.

We ought not to define a democracy as some do, who say simply, that it is a government where the supreme power is lodged in the people; for even in oligarchies the supreme power is in the majority. Nor should they define an oligarchy a government where the supreme power is in the hands of a few:

For let us suppose the number of a people to be thirteen hundred, and that of these one thousand were rich; who would not permit the three hundred poor to have any share in the government? Although they were free, and their equal in everything else, no one would say that this government was a democracy.

In like manner, if the poor, when few in number, should acquire the power over the rich, though more than themselves, no one would say that this was an oligarchy; nor this, when the rest who are rich have no share in the administration. We should rather say that a democracy is when the supreme power is in the hands of the freemen; an oligarchy, when it is in the hands of the rich. It happens indeed that in the one case the many will possess it, in the other the few; because there are many poor and few rich.

GO ON TO THE NEXT PAGE.

24. The author indicates that many forms of government exist because:

A. each form arose from essentially an oligarchy or democracy.
B. there are many forms of magistracies, since they control governments.
C. each state is made up of many kinds of citizens, which governments are meant to serve.
D. each state consists of a great number of parts.

25. If the power of a state were to be distributed according to the beauty of its citizens, the state would be:

A. a republic.
B. an aristocracy.
C. a democracy.
D. an oligarchy.

26. Which of the following statements, if true, would most *weaken* the author's concept of governance?

A. A democracy is a state where the poor are invested with ruling power, and an oligarchy is a state where noble families are invested with ruling power.
B. A democracy is a state where the poor are invested with ruling power, and an oligarchy is a state where the freemen are invested with ruling power.
C. A democracy is a state where noble families are invested with ruling power, and an oligarchy is a state where the poor are invested with ruling power.
D. A democracy is a state where noble families are invested with ruling power, and an oligarchy is a state where the beautiful are invested with ruling power.

27. The main idea of the passage is that:

A. government is a just and fair form of social contract.
B. out of two integral forms of government come all other forms.
C. as there are various kinds of people in society, there are various forms of government.
D. governments are some variant of two essential forms, determined by the size of the ruling party.

28. The author of the passage would probably agree with each of the following statements about government EXCEPT:

A. A democracy occurs when the supreme power is lodged in the people.
B. An oligarchy is like a discordant melody.
C. Several forms of government derive from the oligarchic form.
D. If the poor acquired power over the rich, then a democracy could possibly form.

———————————————

GO ON TO THE NEXT PAGE.

Passage VI (Questions 29 - 34)

The first means of making the rural school a social center is through the course of study. It is here that the introduction of nature-study into our rural schools would be especially helpful.

This nature-study when properly followed approves itself both to educators and to farmers. It is a pedagogical principle recognized by every modern teacher that in education it is necessary to consider the environment of the child, so that the school may not be to him "a thing remote and foreign." The value of nature-study is recognized not only in thus making possible an intelligent study of the country child's environment, but in teaching a love of nature, in giving habits of correct observation, and in preparing for the more fruitful study of science in later years. Our best farmers are also coming to see that nature-study in the rural schools is a necessity, because it will tend to give a knowledge of the laws that govern agriculture, because it will teach the children to love the country, because it will show the possibilities of living an intellectual life upon the farm.

Nature-study, therefore, will have a very direct influence in bringing the child into close touch with the whole life of the farm community.

But it is not so much a matter of introducing new studies—the old studies can be taught in such a way as to make them seem vital and human. Take, for instance, geography. It used to be approached from the standpoint of the solar system. It now begins with the schoolhouse and the pupils' homes, and works outward from the things that the child sees and knows to the things that it must imagine. History, writing, reading, the sciences, and even other subjects can be taught so as to connect them vitally and definitely with the life of the farm community.

A second way of making the rural school a social center is through the social activities of the pupils. This means that the pupils as a body can co-operate for certain purposes, and that this co-operation will not only secure some good results of an immediate character, results that can be seen and appreciated by everyone, but that it will teach the spirit of co-operation—and there is hardly anything more needed today in rural life than this spirit of co-operation.

The schools can perform no better service than in training young people to work together for common ends. In this work such things as special day programs, as for Arbor Day, Washington's Birthday, Pioneer Day; the holding of various school exhibitions; the preparation of exhibits for county fairs, and similar endeavors, are useful and are being carried out in many of our rural schools.

But the best example of this work is a plan that is being used in the state of Maine, and is performed through the agency of what is called a School Improvement League. The purposes of the league are: (1) to improve school grounds and buildings; (2) to furnish suitable reading-matter for pupils and people; (3) to provide works of art for schoolrooms. There are three forms of the league, the local leagues organized in each school; the town leagues, whose membership consists of the officers of the local leagues; and a state league, whose members are delegates from the town leagues and members of the local leagues who hold school diplomas. Any pupil, teacher, school officer, or any other citizen may join the league on payment of the dues.

A third method is through co-operation between the home and the school, between the teacher and pupils on one side, and parents and taxpayers on the other side. Parents sometimes complain that the average school is a sort of mill, or machine, into which their children are placed and turned out just so fast, and in just such condition. But if this is the case, it is partly the fault of the parents who do not keep in close enough touch with the work of the school… There must be the closest co-operation between the home and school. How can this co-operation be brought about?

GO ON TO THE NEXT PAGE.

29. Which of the following findings best supports the author's belief that rural schools should become social centers?

A. Rural schools are not as strong as they should be in history, writing, reading, the sciences and other subjects.
B. Students in rural schools are drifting from the life of farm community.
C. Rural schools are like machines.
D. The School Improvement League requires schools to become social centers.

30. The author of the passage would probably veto most strongly a federal law that:

A. prohibits the rural schools from shortening the total number of school days per year.
B. requires parents of students to visit the rural schools on a periodic basis.
C. assigns to rural schools additional funding for art.
D. grants teachers the right to keep the progress of students private from parents to protect students.

31. The existence of which of the following phenomenon would most strongly challenge the information in the passage?

A. A rural school on the social center paradigm that fosters competition.
B. A graduate of the social center paradigm who abandons farm life.
C. Nature-study produces students who are averse to collaboration.
D. Parents stop sending their children to rural schools on the social center paradigm.

32. According to the passage, which of the following items is(are) values of social centers?

  I.   Correct observation.
  II.   Immediate improvement.
  III. Quality of buildings.

A. I only
B. II only
C. I and III only
D. I, II and III

33. The passage suggests that the cooperation between the home and school is brought about by:

A. Parents visiting the schools often. The teacher knowing more about the home life of her pupils, and the parents knowing far more about the school.
B. Joint meetings of teachers and school officers.
C. The teacher knowing more about the home life of her pupils, and the students knowing far more about the school.
D. Joint meetings of students and school officers.

34. The author most probably advocates each of the following EXCEPT:

A. New studies in the nature-study paradigm over old studies.
B. Teaching correct observation of nature.
C. Preparing students for the study of science.
D. Fostering a foundation of intellectual thinking.

GO ON TO THE NEXT PAGE.

Passage VII (Questions 35 - 40)

Perhaps the most ingenious, as well as the most natural looking product, is the "cultured pearl." This is really natural pearl on much of its exterior, but artificial within and at the back. In order to bring about this result the Japanese, who originated the present commercial product, but who probably borrowed the original idea from the Chinese, call to their assistance the pearl oyster itself.

The oysters are gently opened, small hemispherical discs of mother-of-pearl are introduced between shell and mantle and the oyster replanted. The foreign material is coated by the oyster with true pearly layers as usual, and after several years a sufficiently thick accumulation of pearly layers is thus deposited on the nucleus so that the oyster may be gathered and opened and the cultured pearl removed by sawing it out from the shell to which it has become attached. To the base is then neatly cemented a piece of mother-of-pearl to complete a nearly spherical shape, and the portions of the surface that have not been covered with true pearl are then polished. The product, when set in a proper pearl mounting, is quite convincing and really beautiful…

It is frequently very good however, and for uses that do not demand exposure of the whole surface of the pearl, the cultured pearl supplies a substitute for genuine pearls of moderate quality and price. The back parts of the cultured pearl, being only polished mother-of-pearl, have the appearance of the ordinary pearl button, rather than that of true pearl.

Aside from these half artificial cultured pearls, the out and out imitations of pearls that have been most successfully sold are of two general types, first "Roman pearls," and, second, "Indestructible pearls." The Roman pearls are made hollow and afterward wax filled, the Indestructible pearls have solid enamel bases. In both types the pearly appearance is obtained by lining the interior, or coating the exterior, with more or less numerous layers of what is known as "nacre" or sometimes as "essence d'oriente." This is prepared from the scales of a small fish found in the North Sea and in Russia. The scales are removed and treated with certain solutions which remove the silvery powder from the scales. The "nacre" is then prepared from this powder.

The fineness of the pearly effect becomes greater as the preparation ages, so very fine imitations are usually made from old "nacre." The effect is also better the larger the number of successive layers used. The artificial pearl thus resembles the true pearl in the physical causes for the beautiful effect.

In some cases the Roman pearl has a true iridescence which is produced by "burning" colors into the hollow enamel bead. Some of the indestructible pearls are made over beads of opalescent glass, thus imparting a finer effect to the finished product. While the cheaper grades of indestructible pearls have but three or four layers of nacre, some of the fine ones have as many as thirty or more. The earlier indestructible pearls were made with a coating material which was easily affected by heat, or by water, or by perspiration, as a gelatine-like sizing was included in it. The more recent product has a mineral binder which is not thus affected, so that the "pearls" are really about as durable as natural ones, and will at least last a lifetime if used with proper care.

Like fine natural pearls, the fine imitations should be wiped after use and carefully put away. They should also be restrung occasionally, as should real pearls both to prevent loss by the breaking of the string and because the string becomes soiled after a time, and this hurts the appearance of the jewel.

GO ON TO THE NEXT PAGE.

35. The overall theme of the passage is that:

A. imitation pearls are rather difficult to detect.
B. the distinction between natural and artificial pearls is difficult to make.
C. imitation pearls have several classes and means of detection.
D. pearls can be produced naturally or artificially.

36. According to the passage, how do cultured pearls and natural pearls compare?

A. The time during which the oyster forms a cultured pearl is greater than is required for the growth of a large natural pearl.
B. The number of layers of pearly material is greater in the cultured pearl than the number of layers of a natural pearl.
C. The appearance of the cultured pearl is never equal to that of a fine true pearl.
D. More scales of small North Sea fish are required to make a cultured pearl then those required to make a natural pearl.

37. Suppose a pearl collector wanted to distinguish Roman pearls from contemporary Indestructible pearls. How could the collector make this clear and unmistakable distinction?

A. Heat the two pearls.
B. Look for nacre on Roman pearls.
C. Use a magnifying glass.
D. Put the pearls in a glass of water.

38. How would a collector estimate the age of an imitation pearl?

A. Bisect the pearl and count the number of pearly layers.
B. Look for signs of dirt on the pearl, inside the pearl where the string passes, or on the string itself.
C. Apply a force-measuring instrument to its surface to evaluate durability.
D. Bisect the pearl and count the number of opalescent glass layers.

39. The article from which this passage derives would most likely appear in:

A. a journal for gem collectors.
B. a government report on the pearl trade.
C. an editorial in a trade journal for jewelry.
D. a newspaper op-ed piece.

40. One can infer that the properties of imitation pearls differ from those of natural pearls in each of the following ways EXCEPT:

A. specific gravity.
B. degree of hardness.
C. degree of iridescence.
D. magnified surface characteristics.

STOP.   IF YOU FINISH BEFORE TIME IS CALLED, CHECK YOUR WORK. YOU MAY GO BACK TO ANY QUESTION IN THIS TEST.

STOP.

Verbal Reasoning Test 6

Time: 60 Minutes
Questions 1 - 40

VERBAL REASONING

DIRECTIONS: There are seven passages in the Verbal Reasoning test. Each passage is followed by five to seven questions. Pace yourself and select the one best answer to each question.

Passage I (Questions 1 - 5)

The methods of control which are applicable to general milk supplies are based on the following foundations: (1) the exclusion of all bacterial life, as far as practicable, at the time the milk is drawn, and the subsequent storage of the same at temperatures unfavorable for the growth of the organisms that do gain access; (2) the removal of the bacteria, wholly or in part, after they have once gained access.

The two watch words which are of the utmost importance to the milk dealer are cleanliness and cold. If the milk is properly drawn from the animal in a clean manner and is immediately and thoroughly chilled, the dealer has little to fear as to his product. Whenever serious difficulties do arise, attributable to bacterial changes, it is because negligence has been permitted in one or both directions….

It is of course not practical to take all of these precautions to which reference has been made in the securing of large supplies of market milk for city use, but great improvement over existing conditions could be secured if the public would demand a better supervision of this important food article. Boards of health in our larger cities are awakening to the importance of this question and are becoming increasingly active in the matter of better regulations and the enforcement of the same.

Numerous attempts have been made to find some chemical substance that could be added to milk which would preserve it without interfering with its nutritive properties, but as a general rule a substance that is toxic enough to destroy or inhibit the growth of bacterial life exerts a prejudicial effect on the tissues of the body. The use of chemicals, such as carbolic acid, mercury salts and mineral acids, that are able to entirely destroy all life, is of course excluded, except when milk is preserved for analytical purposes; but a number of milder substances are more or less extensively employed, although the statutes of practically all states forbid their use.

Heat has long been used as a preserving agent. Milk has been scalded or cooked to keep it from time immemorial. Heat may be used at different temperatures, and when so applied exerts a varying effect, depending upon temperature employed… If milk is heated for some minutes to 160° F, it acquires a cooked taste… All methods of preservation by heat rest, however, upon the application of the heat under the following conditions:

1. A temperature above the maximum growing-point (105°-115° F) and below the thermal death-point (130°-140° F) will prevent further growth, and consequently fermentative action;

2. A temperature above the thermal death-point destroys bacteria, and thereby stops all changes. This temperature varies, however, with the condition of the bacteria, and for spores is much higher than for vegetative forms.

GO ON TO THE NEXT PAGE.

When milk, but more especially cream, is heated to 140° F or above, it becomes thinner in consistency or "body," a condition which is due to a change in the grouping of the fat globules…. Heating milk causes the soluble lime salts to be precipitated, and as the curdling of milk by rennet (in cheese-making) is dependent upon the presence of these salts, their absence in heated milks greatly retards the action of rennet.

1. What is the main idea of the passage?

A. Milk is not prepared well enough for human consumption.
B. More methods must be discovered to prepare milk for human consumption.
C. Milk safety begins with bacterial control.
D. Many methods exist to treat milk for human consumption.

2. The passage implies that one hazard of preparing milk for consumption could be:

A. overheating, which creates poor taste.
B. forming too many fat globules.
C. introducing viruses.
D. poisoning by mercury salts.

3. According to the passage, which of the following statements about the growth of bacteria is most accurate?

A. A maximum temperature exists that prevents growth.
B. Just because bacterial organisms stop dividing does not mean they are dead.
C. Bacteria in milk exist primarily in spore forms.
D. Above the maximum growing-point, bacteria does not cause milk to change.

4. The author would disagree with each of the following statements EXCEPT:

A. Heated milk is not adequate for making cheese.
B. Violations of cleanliness or cold preservation contribute mostly to bacterial changes in milk.
C. Milk should always be kept chilled once drawn from the animal until consumption.
D. People have little say in the control of milk.

5. The author would most likely agree with which of the following statements about treating milk?

A. Mild forms of poisons are no longer used in the treatment of milk.
B. Treating milk with heat arose after the discovery of chemical treatment.
C. Treating milk with chemicals affects its lime salt content.
D. Milk dealers who use clean and cooling methods for drawing milk rarely encounter bacterial problems.

GO ON TO THE NEXT PAGE.

Passage II (Questions 6 - 10)

How shall I make it clear to you the extreme difficulty which we in Flatland experience in recognizing one another's configuration?

All beings in Flatland, animate and inanimate, no matter what their form, present to our view the same, or nearly the same, appearance, viz. that of a straight Line. How then can one be distinguished from another, where all appear the same?

The answer is threefold. The first means of recognition is the sense of hearing; which with us is far more highly developed than with you, and which enables us not only to distinguish by the voice of our personal friends, but even to discriminate between different classes, at least so far as concerns the three lowest orders, the Equilateral, the Square, and the Pentagon--for the Isosceles I take no account.

But as we ascend the social scale, the process of discriminating and being discriminated by hearing increases in difficulty, partly because voices are assimilated, partly because the faculty of voice-discrimination is a plebeian virtue not much developed among the Aristocracy. And wherever there is any danger of imposture we cannot trust to this method. Amongst our lowest orders, the vocal organs are developed to a degree more than correspondent with those of hearing, so that an Isosceles can easily feign the voice of a Polygon, and, with some training, that of a Circle himself. A second method is therefore more commonly resorted to…

If Fog were non-existent, all lines would appear equally and indistinguishably clear; and this is actually the case in those unhappy countries in which the atmosphere is perfectly dry and transparent

Suppose I see two individuals approaching whose rank I wish to ascertain. They are, we will suppose, a Merchant and a Physician, or in other words, an Equilateral Triangle and a Pentagon, respectively; how am I to distinguish them?

It will be obvious, to every child in Spaceland who has touched the threshold of Geometrical Studies, [where a polygon's interior angle is equal to $(180n - 360)/n$] that, if I can bring my eye so that its glance may bisect an angle (A) of the approaching stranger, my view will lie as it were evenly between the two sides that are next to me (viz. CA and AB), so that I shall contemplate the two impartially, and both will appear of the same size.

Now in the case of the Merchant, what shall I see? I shall see a straight line DAE, in which the middle point (A) will be very bright because it is nearest to me; but on either side the line will shade away rapidly to dimness, because the sides AC and AB recede rapidly into the fog and what appear to me as the Merchant's extremities, viz. D and E, will be very dim indeed…

According to his account, my unfortunate Ancestor… who indeed obtained, shortly before his decease, four out of seven votes from the Sanitary and Social Board for passing him into the class of the Equal-sided… being afflicted with rheumatism, and in the act of being felt by a Polygon, by one sudden start accidentally transfixed the Great Man through the diagonal and thereby, partly in consequence of his long imprisonment and degradation, and partly because of the moral shock which pervaded the whole of my Ancestor's relations, threw back our family a degree and a half in their ascent towards better things.

The result was that in the next generation the family brain was registered at only 58 degrees, and not till the lapse of five generations was the lost ground recovered, the full 60 degrees attained, and the Ascent from the Isosceles finally achieved.

GO ON TO THE NEXT PAGE.

6. Which natural sense, if greatly enhanced, would be most effective in preventing the occurrence of impostors?

A. Movement.
B. Texture.
C. Smell.
D. Hearing.

7. According to the passage, which of the following is most likely to be true about how various beings appear in Fog?

    I.   The Circle will always appear as a straight line with a bright center.

    II.   The Square will always appear as a straight line with a bright center.

    III.   All Polygons always appear as a straight line with a bright center

A. I only
B. II only
C. II and III only
D. I, II, and III

8. According to the passage, how would the Physician appear?

A. A line with a bright center, but the lines of its sides recede less rapidly in the fog and will thus appear less dim as those of the Merchant.
B. A line with a bright center, but the lines of its sides recede more rapidly in the fog and will thus appear dimmer than those of the Merchant.
C. A line with a dimmer center, while the lines of its sides will appear as dim as those of the Merchant.
D. A line with a brighter center, while the lines of its sides will appear as dim as those of the Merchant.

9. A likely title for this written piece is:

A. Geometry in a Flat World.
B. Flatland, the Life.
C. Journey in Spaceland.
D. Hearing and Sight in a Flat World.

10. Suppose a physician were afflicted with rheumatism and his brain was registered at 95 degrees. After five generations making a full recovery, to what degree would his brain return?

A. 97 degrees.
B. 98 degrees.
C. 108 degrees.
D. 120 degrees.

GO ON TO THE NEXT PAGE.

Passage III (Questions 11 - 15)

The great and leading cause of the present state to which the Royal Society is reduced, may be traced to years of misrule to which it has been submitted…

It is known, that by the statutes, the body of the Society have the power of electing, annually, their President, Officers, and Council; and it is also well known, that this is a merely nominal power, and that printed lists are prepared and put into the hands of the members on their entering the room, and thus passed into the balloting box. If these lists were, as in other scientific societies, openly discussed in the Council, and then offered by them as recommendations to the Society, little inconvenience would arise; but the fact is, that they are private nominations by the President, usually without notice, to the Council, and all the supporters of the system which I am criticizing, endeavor to uphold the right of this nomination in the President, and prevent or discourage any alteration.

The Society has, for years, been managed by a party, or coterie, or by whatever other name may be most fit to designate a combination of persons, united by no expressed compact or written regulations, but who act together from a community of principles. That each individual has invariably supported all the measures of the party, is by no means the case; and whilst instances of opposition amongst them have been very rare, a silent resignation to circumstances has been the most usual mode of meeting measures they disapproved.

The great object of this, as of all other parties, has been to maintain itself in power, and to divide, as far as it could, all the good things amongst its members. It has usually consisted of persons of very moderate talent, who have had the prudence, whenever they could, to associate with themselves other members of greater ability, provided these latter would not oppose the system, and would thus lend to it the sanction of their name. The party have always praised each other most highly—have invariably opposed all improvements in the Society, all change in the mode of management; and have maintained, that all those who wished for any alteration were factious; and, when they discovered any symptoms of independence and inquiry breaking out in any member of the Council, they have displaced him as soon as they decently could.

Of the arguments employed by those who support the system of management by which the Royal Society is governed, I shall give a few samples: refutation is rendered quite unnecessary— juxtaposition is alone requisite. If any member, seeing an improper appointment in contemplation, or any abuse in the management of the affairs of the Society… raise a voice against it, the ready answer is, Why should you interfere? it may not be quite the thing you approve; but it is no affair of yours.

If, on the other hand, it does relate to himself, the reply is equally ready. It is immediately urged.

The question is of a personal nature; you are the last person who ought to bring it forward; you are yourself interested. If any member of the Society, feeling annoyed at the neglect, or hurt by the injuries or insults of the Council, show signs of remonstrance, it is immediately suggested to him that he is irritated, and ought to wait until his feelings subside, and he can judge more coolly on the subject; whilst with becoming candor they admit the ill-treatment, but urge forbearance.

If, after an interval, when reflection has had ample time to operate, the offense seems great as at first, or the insult appears unmitigated by any circumstances on which memory can dwell,—if it is then brought forward, the immediate answer is, The affair is out of date—the thing is gone by—it is too late to call in question a transaction so long past. Thus, if a man is interested personally, he is unfit to question an abuse; if he is not, is it probable that he will question it? and if, notwithstanding this, he do so, then he is to be accounted a meddler.

GO ON TO THE NEXT PAGE.

11. Each of the following statements is supported in the passage EXCEPT:

A. Silent resignation is a common mode of disapproval.
B. Individuals have supported all the measures of the party.
C. Remonstrance is not well tolerated by the Council.
D. Even after an interval of time has passed will a complaint be discredited by the Council.

12. According to the author, a better election system would consist of:

A. private nominations by the President.
B. a symposium to review nominees.
C. open discussion by the Society.
D. a forum of discussion led by the President.

13. According to the passage, after a member of the Society cools off and brings forth an offense again, the reaction to him would be:

A. Recognition, since he has waited for an interval.
B. Acceptance, since he has calmed down.
C. Disregard, since he was irritated.
D. Dismissal, since the offense has expired.

14. The existence of which of the following procedures would most strongly challenge the information in the passage?

A. The Society's consideration of an offense by a member of the Council.
B. The party opposing all improvements to the Society.
C. Open reception to the complaint of a member of the Society about an improper appointment.
D. The Council and the Society working in cooperation.

15. The passage implies that the party is open to suggestions by the Society under which circumstances?

A. After the member of Society waits a certain length of time.
B. When the Society as a group submits a written appeal to the party.
C. After the member of Society retracts his complaint.
D. None. The party stonewalls members of the Society.

GO ON TO THE NEXT PAGE.

Passage IV (Questions 16 - 22)

For play is necessary for relaxation, and relaxation pleasant, as it is a medicine for that uneasiness which arises from labor. It is admitted also that a happy life must be an honorable one, and a pleasant one too, since happiness consists in both these; and we all agree that music is one of the most pleasing things, whether alone or accompanied with a voice; as Musseus says, "Music's the sweetest joy of man;" for which reason it is justly admitted into every company and every happy life, as having the power of inspiring joy.

So that from this any one may suppose that it is necessary to instruct young persons in it; for all those pleasures which are harmless are not only conducive to the final end of life, but serve also as relaxations; and, as men are but rarely in the attainment of that final end, they often cease from their labor and apply to amusement, with no further view than to acquire the pleasure attending it.

It is therefore useful to enjoy such pleasures as these. There are some persons who make play and amusement their end, and probably that end has some pleasure annexed to it, but not what should be; but while men seek the one they accept the other for it; because there is some likeness in human actions to the end; for the end is pursued for the sake of nothing else that attends it; but for itself only; and pleasures like these are sought for, not on account of what follows them, but on account of what has gone before them, as labor and grief; for which reason they seek for happiness in these sort of pleasures; and that this is the reason any one may easily perceive.

That music should be pursued, not on this account only, but also as it is very serviceable during the hours of relaxation from labor, probably no one doubts; we should also inquire whether besides this use it may not also have another of nobler nature—and we ought not only to partake of the common pleasure arising from it (which all have the sensation of, for music naturally gives pleasure, therefore the use of it is agreeable to all ages and all dispositions); but also to examine if it tends anything to improve our manners and our souls. And this will be easily known if we feel our dispositions any way influenced thereby; and that they are so is evident from many other instances, as well as the music at the Olympic games; and this confessedly fills the soul with enthusiasm; but enthusiasm is an affection of the soul which strongly agitates the disposition.

Besides, all those who hear any imitations sympathize therewith; and this when they are conveyed even without rhythm or verse. Moreover, as music is one of those things which are pleasant, and as virtue itself consists in rightly enjoying, loving, and hating, it is evident that we ought not to learn or accustom ourselves to anything so much as to judge right and rejoice in honorable manners and noble actions.

But anger and mildness, courage and modesty, and their contraries, as well as all other dispositions of the mind, are most naturally imitated by music and poetry; which is plain by experience, for when we hear these our very soul is altered; and he who is affected either with joy or grief by the imitation of any objects, is in very nearly the same situation as if he was affected by the objects themselves; thus, if any person is pleased with seeing a statue of any one on no other account but its beauty, it is evident that the sight of the original from whence it was taken would also be pleasing; now it happens in the other senses there is no imitation of manners; that is to say, in the touch and the taste; in the objects of sight, a very little; for these are merely representations of things, and the perceptions which they excite are in a manner common to all.

GO ON TO THE NEXT PAGE.

16. According to the passage, when does enjoying pleasure become useful?

A. When it is sought after a day of work with no further consideration than to enjoy the pleasure itself.
B. When music accompanies it.
C. When the object of enjoyment is imitated.
D. When we feel our dispositions.

17. The author would most likely disagree with which of the following statements:

A. Music gives pleasure naturally.
B. Harmful pleasures are not necessarily relaxing.
C. Music is best pursued when enjoyment of it is the sole reason for hearing it.
D. The pleasure of an apple cannot be imitated.

18. The tone of the author is best described as:

A. high-flown.
B. erudite.
C. trite.
D. enthusiastic.

19. The passage implies that a person who lives a life of virtue and happiness must:

A. pursue pleasure, preferably in the form of music and poetry.
B. live by courage and modesty, mildness and anger when appropriate.
C. live by enthusiasm, courage and modesty, and seek pleasure after a day of labor.
D. be pleasant and honorable, and enjoy what should be enjoyed, and hate what should be hated.

20. The passage suggests that the author would agree with each of the following statements EXCEPT:

A. A sculptor who molds a beautiful sculpture can experience the same pleasure as another sculptor who molds a similar sculpture.
B. A child's fear of a costume of a large bear is as legitimate as his fear of a real bear.
C. A sculptor and painter looking at the same sculpture can share the same level of enjoyment.
D. A chef's enjoyment of a soup can be as pleasing as his enjoyment of a different soup.

21. This passage would most likely appear in which format?

A. poetry journal.
B. health and wellness publication.
C. newspaper editorial.
D. creative writing journal.

22. The most likely title of this article is:

A. The Happiness of Art
B. Music and Relaxation
C. Enjoy Life the Right Way
D. Happiness and Virtue

GO ON TO THE NEXT PAGE.

Passage V (Questions 23 - 28)

The coat of arms of Mexico has its origin in the distant past. General Lew Wallace says in his historical romance the Fair God: "The site of the city of Tenochtitlan was chosen by the gods. In the southwestern border of Lake Tezcuco, one morning in 1300, a wandering tribe of Aztecs saw an eagle perched, with outspread wings, upon a cactus, and holding a serpent in its talons. At a word from their priests, they took possession of the marsh and there stayed their migration and founded the city; such is the tradition."

In the early days of stamps, most countries made their own and they were, in some degree, an indication of the artistic progress, or want of it, in a country. But we have changed all that and today all effort seems to be directed toward producing artistic and attractive stamps. Sometimes this is due to national pride and occasionally it is intended to draw attention to the resources and natural wonders of a country. But too often, we fear, these picture stamps are produced merely with a view to their ready salability to collectors.

More frequently than not, these brilliant labels are the product of a distant country and are no longer indicative of the artistic status of the country by which they are issued. Indeed, the wilds of Africa, the distant islands of the Pacific and the tumultuous republics of Central America far outshine the cultured countries of the old world in their postal stationery.

The majority of stamps bear a portrait, usually that of a sovereign. The stamps of our own country present a portrait gallery of our great and heroic dead, for by law the faces of the living may not appear on our stamps or money. This is the reverse of the rule in monarchical countries, where the portrait of the reigning sovereign usually adorns the postal issues.

Many nations have used their coats of arms as appropriate decorations for their postal issues. On the five shilling stamps of Malta we find the Maltese cross, emblem of the Knights of St. John and reminiscent of the crusades.

New Foundland, Nova Scotia and New Brunswick have adorned their stamps with the heraldic rose, thistle and shamrock of the British Empire.

The stamps of Rhodesia and the Congo Free State depict the advance of civilization. Egypt has her sphinx and pyramids; Greece an artistic series of pictures of her famous statues and ruins. Fiji shows a pirogue, the native canoe, rudely shaped from a tree trunk and hollowed out by fire. Labuan has a piratical-looking native dhow.

Very familiar to collectors are the camel of Obock and the Soudan, the Llama of Peru, and the sacred quetzal of Guatemala. In other countries only inscriptions are used. This is especially the case with the Native States of India, in some of which as many as four languages are said to be employed on one stamp

Stereotypes or electrotypes of single stamps are called cliches. In making up a plate it sometimes happens that a cliche is placed upside down. The result, after printing, is a stamp in that position. Like all oddities these are prized by stamp collectors. The method of cancellation used in Afghanistan is crude but effective. It consists in cutting or tearing a piece out of the stamp.

GO ON TO THE NEXT PAGE.

23. The main argument of the passage is that:

A. Stamps represent the artistic progress of the country that made it.
B. Stamps are no longer indicative of the artistic status of the country by which they are issued.
C. Stamps are the focus of the artistic efforts of a nation.
D. Stamps depict aspects of achievement for a given nation.

24. The author is most concerned about which of the following driving forces for the production of stamps?

A. strong pride of a nation.
B. appeal to collectors.
C. artistic expression of a society.
D. promotion of natural resources.

25. According to the passage, a stamp bearing only inscriptions might be considered each of the following EXCEPT:

A. unpopular with collectors, probably because of their inability to read them.
B. valuable, because stamps of this nature are rare.
C. interesting for their crude and curious designs.
D. informative, because they may reveal which cultures coexist.

26. The author would expect the designs of stamps to suggest many things, EXCEPT the:

A. power of nations.
B. technology of civilizations.
C. prosperous future of a society.
D. scenic grandeur of a country.

27. Which of the following examples would best describe a contemporary stamp?

A. A stamp made in Brazil depicting life on the Amazon River.
B. A late issue of the Eiffel Tower made in Paris.
C. A late issue from the Tonga islands but made in London.
D. A stamp depicting a coat of arms with the portrait of a king.

28. The discussion of General Lew Wallace's Fair God suggests that as men love to trace their descent back to some past greatness:

A. civilizations seek to associate a divine animal with their prosperity.
B. nations take pride in their foundation at the hands of a religious leader.
C. civilizations trace their descent back to a symbol of divinity.
D. nations delight to associate the gods with their origin.

_____

GO ON TO THE NEXT PAGE.

Passage VI (Questions 29 - 34)

Along with good tillage must go crop-rotation and good drainage. A supply of organic matter will prevent heavy rains from washing away the soil and carrying away plant food. Drainage will aid good tillage in allowing air to circulate between the soil particles and in arranging plant food so that plants can use it.

But we must add humus, or vegetable matter, to the soil. You remember that the virgin soils contained a great deal of vegetable matter and plant food, but by the continuous growing of crops like wheat, corn, and cotton, and by constant shallow tillage, both humus and plant food have been used up. Consequently much of our cultivated soil today is hard and dead.

There are three ways of adding humus and plant food to this lifeless land: the first way is to apply barnyard manure (to adopt this method means that livestock raising must be a part of all farming); the second way is to adopt rotation of crops, and frequently to plow under crops like clover and cowpeas; the third way is to apply commercial fertilizers.

He should understand also that liquid manure is of more value than solid, because that important plant food, nitrogen, is found almost wholly in the liquid portion. Some of the phosphoric acid and considerable amounts of the potash are also found in the liquid manure. Hence economy requires that none of this escape either by leakage or by fermentation. Sometimes one can detect the smell of ammonia in the stable. This ammonia is formed by the decomposition of the liquid manure, and its loss should be checked by sprinkling some floats, acid phosphate, or muck over the stable floor.

Many farmers find it desirable to buy fertilizers to use with the manure made on the farm. In this case it is helpful to understand the composition, source, and availability of the various substances composing commercial fertilizers. The three most valuable things in commercial fertilizers are nitrogen, potash, and phosphoric acid.

The nitrogen is obtained from (1) nitrate of soda mined in Chile, (2) ammonium sulphate, a by-product of the gas works, (3) dried blood and other by-products of the slaughter-houses, and (4) cotton-seed meal. Nitrate of soda is soluble in water and may therefore be washed away before being used by plants. For this reason it should be applied in small quantities and at intervals of a few weeks.

Potash is obtained in Germany, where it is found in several forms. It is put on the market as muriate of potash, sulphate of potash, kainite, which contains salt as an impurity, and in other impure forms. Potash is found also in unleached wood ashes.

Phosphoric acid is found in various rocks of Tennessee, Florida, and South Carolina, and also to a large extent in bones. The rocks or bones are usually treated with sulphuric acid. This treatment changes the phosphoric acid into a form ready for plant use.

These three kinds of plant food are ordinarily all that we need to supply. In some cases, however, lime has to be added. Besides being a plant food itself, lime helps most soils by improving the structure of the grains; by sweetening the soil, thereby aiding the little living germs called bacteria; by hastening the decay of organic matter; and by setting free the potash that is locked up in the soil.

GO ON TO THE NEXT PAGE.

29. According to the passage, which of the following describes complete soil cultivation?

A. Barnyard liquid manure with crop-rotation, tillage and drainage.
B. Kainite, dried blood and byproducts, bone treated with sulphuric acid, and lime with shallow tillage, drainage and crop rotation.
C. Florida rocks treated with sulphuric acid, cotton-seed meal, and wood ashes with deep tillage, crop-rotation, and drainage.
D. Soda from Chile, muriate of potash, and lime with tillage, crop-rotation and drainage.

30. The author would most likely agree with which of the following statements?

A. Excellent nitrogen sources are found in Germany.
B. The decay of organic matter is not beneficial for the soil.
C. Corn and cotton use up soil nutrients faster than many other crops.
D. The smell of ammonia in the table is unnatural.

31. As implied by the passage, how would a farmer improve the quality of soil year after year?

A. Apply good tillage and crop-rotation, drain well, and add humus and plant food.
B. Grow wheat in virgin soil with tillage and drainage.
C. Use lime and nitrogen with crop-rotation, deep tillage, and dried blood
D. Use shallow tillage in times of excess rain, along with phosphoric acid, nitrogen, and potash.

32. Which method of fertilizing would most likely incur the *greatest* cost?

A. Adding phosphoric acid from South Carolina rocks.
B. Plow under cowpeas.
C. Applying barnyard fertilizer.
D. Adding cotton-seed meal.

33. During the rainy season, a prudent farmer would take which action?

A. Apply lime and extra kainite.
B. Apply ammonium sulphate in small quantities at various intervals.
C. Apply extra nitrogen in each application in the form of cotton-seed meal.
D. Apply less drainage so as to minimize nutrients washing away.

34. Given that a plot of land contains dead soil, how would the author propose to revive it?

A. Remove the bad soil, add solid barnyard manure mixed with lime, then apply drainage and crop-rotation with tillage.
B. Remove the bad soil, add fresh soil mixed with liquid manure, then apply drainage and crop-rotation with tillage.
C. Remove the bad soil, add humus and plant food, then apply crop-rotation with tillage.
D. Remove the bad soil, add ammonium sulphate and kainite, then apply drainage and crop-rotation with tillage.

GO ON TO THE NEXT PAGE.

Passage VII (Questions 35 - 40)

The strength, courage, and majestic deportment of this noble animal has gained him the regal titles of monarch of the forest and king of beasts. Ancient heralds selected the figure of the lion as symbolic of command, strength, power, courage, and other qualities attributed to that animal.

Armorists have introduced lions to denote the attributes of majesty, might, and clemency, subduing those that resist, and sparing those that yield to authority. The lion has been depicted in every attitude which could by any means be construed into a compliment to the person the sovereign delighted to honor, by raising him to a rank that enabled him to bear arms. Was it a warrior, who, though victorious, was still engaged in struggling with the foes of his sovereign, the lion rampant was considered a proper emblem of the hero. The warrior having overcome his enemies in the field, yet retaining his military command for the safety and honor of his country, was typified by the lion standing guardant.

The allegorical designs emblazoned on the standards, shields, and armor of the Greeks and Romans-the White Horse of the Saxons, the Raven of the Danes, and the Lion of the Normans, may all be termed heraldic devices; but according to the opinions of Camden, Spelman, and other high authorities, hereditary arms of families were first introduced at the commencement of the twelfth century. When numerous armies engaged in the expeditions to the Holy Land, consisting of the troops of twenty different nations, they were obliged to adopt some ensign or mark in order to marshal the vassals under the banners of the various leaders.

The regulation of the symbols whereby the Sovereigns and Lords of Europe should be distinguished, all of whom were ardent in maintaining the honor of the several nations to which they belonged, was a matter of great nicety, and it was properly entrusted to the Heralds who invented signs of honor which could not be construed into offense, and made general regulations for their display on the banners and shields of the chiefs of the different nations.

The passion for military fame which prevailed at this period led to the introduction of mock battles, called Tournaments. Here the Knights appeared with the Heraldic honors conferred upon them for deeds of prowess in actual battle. All were emulous of such distinctions. The subordinate followers appeared with the distinctive arms of their Lord, with the addition of some mark denoting inferiority.

Honorable ordinaries were the original marks of distinction bestowed by sovereigns on subjects that had become eminent for their services, either in the councilor the field of battle. Volumes have been written upon the origin and form of the honorable ordinaries.

Arms of Dominion or Sovereignty were properly the arms of the kings or sovereigns of the territories they govern, which were also regarded as the arms of the State. Thus the Lions of England and the Russian Eagle were the arms of the Kings of England and the Emperors of Russia, and could not properly be altered by a change of dynasty.

Arms of Pretension were those of kingdoms, provinces, or territories to which a prince or lord had some claim, and which he added to his own, though the kingdoms or territories were governed by a foreign king or lord: thus the Kings of England for many ages quartered the arms of France in their escutcheon as the descendants of Edward III, who claimed that kingdom, in right of his mother, a French princess.

Arms of Community are those of bishoprics, cities, universities, academies, societies, and corporate bodies.

Arms of Concession were arms granted by sovereigns as the reward of virtue, valor, or extraordinary service. All arms granted to subjects were originally conceded by the Sovereign.

GO ON TO THE NEXT PAGE.

35. According to the passage, the author would most likely agree with which statement?

A. Chiefs of nations contributed to the design of their heraldic arms.
B. Heraldic arms were the exclusive domain of knights, chiefs, and sovereigns.
C. Honorable marks of distinction were bestowed primarily for achievements in battle.
D. Heraldic arms never included offensive signs.

36. A sovereign would feel disinclined to bestow the figure of a lion on a person who performed which action?

A. Remaining on the battlefield after the battle has ended.
B. Punishing enemies after they have surrendered.
C. Jailing instigators of an uprising.
D. Parading through a conquered town.

37. Which of the following attributes did not contribute directly to the origination and evolution of heraldry?

A. pomp
B. military fame
C. loyalty to sovereigns
D. extraordinary council

38. Suppose that the King of Spain conquered the Kingdom of Prussia. Which of the following repercussions would most likely occur?

A. The Prussian Arms of Dominion would change.
B. Cities of Prussia would change their Arms of Community.
C. The King of Spain would grant the Arms of Concession to the King of Prussia.
D. The Spanish Arms of Pretension would change.

39. According to the passage, which of the following depict historic uses of emblazoned arms?

    I.   Mark of distinction.
    II.   Device of organization
    III.   Sign of submission.

A. I only
B. III only
C. I and II only
D. I, II, and III

40. Which modern-day practice most nearly captures the purpose and significance of heraldic arms of the past?

A. Emblems representing military squadrons.
B. Coat of arms representing family names.
C. Seals representing presidents of nations.
D. Symbols representing historic events found on currency.

STOP.   IF YOU FINISH BEFORE TIME IS CALLED, CHECK YOUR WORK. YOU MAY GO BACK TO ANY QUESTION IN THIS TEST.

STOP.

Verbal Reasoning Test 7

Time: 60 Minutes
Questions 1 - 40

VERBAL REASONING

DIRECTIONS: There are seven passages in the Verbal Reasoning test. Each passage is followed by five to seven questions. Pace yourself and select the one best answer to each question.

Passage I (Questions 1 - 5)

The essence of feudalism was a gradation of rank, in the nature of caste, based upon fear. The clergy were privileged because the laity believed that they could work miracles, and could dispense something more vital even than life and death. The nobility were privileged because they were resistless in war. Therefore, the nobility could impose all sorts of burdens upon those who were unarmed. During the interval in which society centralized and acquired more and more a modern economic form, the discrepancies in status remained, while commensurately the physical or imaginative force which had once sustained inequality declined, until the social equilibrium grew to be extremely unstable. Add to this that France, under the monarchy, was ill consolidated. The provinces and towns retained the administrative complexity of an archaic age, even to local tariffs. Thus under the monarchy privilege and inequality pervaded every phase of life, and, as the judiciary must be, more or less, the mouthpiece of society, the judiciary came to be the incarnation of caste…

The corvée threw the burden of maintaining the highways on the peasantry by exacting forced labor. It was admittedly the most hateful, the most burdensome, and the most wasteful of all the bad taxes of the time, and Turgot, following the precedent of the Roman Empire, advised instead a general highway impost. The proposed impost in itself was not considerable, and would not have been extraordinarily obnoxious to the privileged classes, but for the principle of equality by which Turgot justified it: "The expenses of government having for their object the interests of all, all should contribute to them; and the more advantages a man has, the more that man should contribute."

…such service had long ceased to be performed, while on the contrary, titles could be bought for money. Hence every wealthy man became a noble when he pleased…

…By this thrust, the privileged classes felt themselves wounded in their vitals, and the Parliament of Paris, the essence of privilege, assumed their defense. To be binding, the edicts had to be registered by the Parliament among the laws of France, and Parliament declined to make registration on the ground that the edicts were unconstitutional, as subversive of the monarchy and of the principle of order. The opinion of the court was long, but a single paragraph gives its purport: "The first rule of justice is to preserve to every one what belongs to him: this rule consists, not only in preserving the rights of property, but still more in preserving those belonging to the person, which arise from the prerogative of birth and of position…

From this rule of law and equity it follows that every system which, under an appearance of humanity and beneficence, would tend to establish between men an equality of duties, and to destroy necessary distinctions, would soon lead to disorder (the inevitable result of equality), and would bring about the overturn of civil society."

GO ON TO THE NEXT PAGE.

This judicial opinion was an enunciation of the archaic law of caste as opposed to the modern law of equality, and the cataclysm of the French Revolution hinged upon the incapacity of the French aristocracy to understand that the environment, which had once made caste a necessity, had yielded to another which made caste an impossibility.

1. Suppose that the nobility enjoyed exemption from taxation. Which of the following statements, if true, would best represent a justification of this exemption by Turgot?

A. Nobles are bound to yield military service without pay.
B. Nobles are privileged and not bound to any service.
C. Taxation without representation is unjust.
D. Nobles comprise the government, and a government cannot tax itself.

2. The passage indicates that the Parliament of Paris believed:

A. equality of duties among citizens preserves civil society.
B. an imbalance between rich and poor exists in every society.
C. positions of privilege is a birthright.
D. the caste system establishes a foundation for society.

3. The author suggests that commoners in France challenged feudalism when they:

A. obtained wealth from economic reform.
B. gained control of provinces and towns.
C. gained access to the judiciary, and discovered that the nobility could not harm them.
D. gained access to weaponry, and discovered that the Church could neither harm nor aid them.

4. The tone of the author can be best described as:

A. neutral.
B. insightful.
C. critical.
D. cynical.

5. Positions of privilege are described as "titles… bought for money." Turgot does not support this practice most likely because it:

A. challenges the principle of order.
B. supports the Parliament of Paris.
C. broadens the gap between rich and poor.
D. transforms the judiciary into a caste.

_____

GO ON TO THE NEXT PAGE.

Passage II (Questions 6 - 12)

It may seem wonderful that language, which is the only method of conveying our conceptions, should, at the same time, be a hindrance to our advancement in philosophy; but the wonder ceases when we consider, that it is seldom studied as the vehicle of truth, but is too frequently esteemed for its own sake, independent of its connection with things…

…every lover of truth will only study a language for the purpose of procuring the wisdom it contains; and will doubtless wish to make his native language the vehicle of it to others. For, since all truth is eternal, its nature can never be altered by transposition, though by this means its dress may be varied, and become less elegant and refined. Perhaps even this inconvenience may be remedied by sedulous cultivation; at least, the particular inability of some, ought not to discourage the well-meant endeavors of others.

Whoever reads the lives of the ancient Heroes of Philosophy, must be convinced that they studied things more than words, and that Truth alone was the ultimate object of their search; and he who wishes to emulate their glory and participate in their wisdom, will study their doctrines more than their language, and value the depth of their understandings far beyond the elegance of their composition. The native charms of Truth will ever be sufficient to allure the truly philosophic mind; and he who has once discovered her retreats will surely endeavor to fix a mark by which they may be detected by others.

But, though the mischief arising from the study of words is prodigious, we must not consider it as the only cause of darkening the splendors of Truth, and obstructing the free diffusion of her light. Different manners and philosophies have equally contributed to banish the goddess from our realms, and to render our eyes offended with her celestial light. Hence we must not wonder that, being indignant at the change, and perceiving the empire of ignorance rising to unbounded dominion, she has retired from the spreading darkness, and concealed herself in the tranquil and divinely lucid regions of mind. For we need but barely survey modern pursuits to be convinced how little they are connected with wisdom. Since, to describe the nature of some particular place, the form, situation and magnitude of a certain city; to trace the windings of a river to its source, or delineate the aspect of a pleasant mountain; to calculate the fineness of the silkworm's threads, and arrange the gaudy colors of butterflies; in short, to pursue matter through its infinite divisions, and wander in its dark labyrinths, is the employment of the philosophy in vogue. But surely the energies of intellect are more worthy our concern than the operations of sense; and the science of universals, permanent and fixed, must be superior to the knowledge of particulars, fleeting and frail…

The design of the following discourse is to bring us to the perception of the beautiful itself, even while connected with a corporeal nature, which must be the great end of all true philosophy and which Plotinus happily obtained. To a genius, indeed, truly modern, with whom the crucible and the air-pump are alone the standards of Truth, such an attempt must appear ridiculous in the extreme…

But here it is requisite to observe that our ascent to this region of Beauty must be made by gradual advances, for, from our association with matter, it is impossible to pass directly, and without a medium, to such transcendent perfection…

It is necessary therefore, that we should become very familiar with the most abstract contemplations; and that our intellectual eye should be strongly irradiated with the light of ideas which precedes the splendors of the beautiful itself…

6. The author suggests that the study of matter:

A. conceals itself in the mind.
B. eludes the philosophers of his day.
C. is similar to the study of Beauty.
D. leads to endless experiments.

7. Which of the following would suggest that the author's concern about the pursuit of Truth is exaggerated?

A. A physicist offers theories on light behavior.
B. A linguist proposes a new philosophy on truth.
C. A psychologist reveals the subconscious meanings of joy.
D. A philosopher creates a new philosophy.

8. Which of the following statements is inconsistent with information in the passage?

A. Language, when used improperly, alters the nature of truth.
B. Matter influences how we discover Beauty.
C. A genius does not bother with the study of details.
D. The study of details can waste intellectual energy

9. The assertion that the "science of universals, permanent and fixed, must be superior to the knowledge of particulars," is:

A. supported by Plotinus.
B. supported by the author's discussion of the perception of Beauty.
C. contradicted by the author's own use of language.
D. contradicted by examples set by the Heroes of Philosophy.

10. Suppose the author uses the metaphor "like the brightness which is seen on the summit of mountains previous to the rising of the sun." This image describes most likely the concept of:

A. Truth, and the process of discovering it.
B. Language, and the process of understanding it.
C. Beauty, and the process of perceiving it.
D. Intellect, and the process of using it.

11. The reference to "the gaudy colors of butterflies" suggests that the author:

A. dislikes frail things.
B. disapproves of nature's wisdom.
C. does not want to spend time defining minutia.
D. has another definition of Beauty.

12. This passage was written most likely for:

A. biologists.
B. philosophers.
C. students.
D. psychologists.

_____

GO ON TO THE NEXT PAGE.

Passage III (Questions 13 - 18)

Near the base of the zone of solution veins are often stored with exceptionally large and valuable ore deposits. This local enrichment of the vein is due to the reconcentration of its metalliferous ores. As the surface of the land is slowly lowered by weathering and running water, the zone of solution is lowered at an equal rate and encroaches constantly on the zone of cementation. The minerals of veins are therefore constantly being dissolved along their upper portions and carried down the fissures by ground water to lower levels, where they are redeposited.

It is to the igneous rocks that we may look for the original source of the metals of veins. Lavas contain minute percentages of various metallic compounds, and no doubt this was the case also with the igneous rocks which formed the original earth crust. By the erosion of the igneous rocks the metals have been distributed among sedimentary strata, and even the sea has taken into solution an appreciable amount of gold and other metals, but in this widely diffused condition they are wholly useless to man. The concentration which has made them available is due to the interaction of many agencies. Earth movements fracturing deeply the rocks of the crust, the intrusion of heated masses, the circulation of underground waters, have all cooperated in the concentration of the metals of mineral veins.

While fissure veins are the most important of mineral veins, the latter term is applied also to any water way which has been filled by similar deposits from solution. Thus in soluble rocks, such as limestones, joints enlarged by percolating water are sometimes filled with metalliferous deposits, as, for example, the lead and zinc deposits of the upper Mississippi valley. Even a porous aquifer may be made the seat of mineral deposits, as in the case of some copper-bearing and silver-bearing sandstones of New Mexico.

The correlation of formations by means of fossils may be explained by the formations now being deposited about the north Atlantic. Lithologically they are extremely various. On the continental shelf of North America limestones of different kinds are forming off Florida, and sandstones and shales from Georgia northward. Separated from them by the deep Atlantic oozes are other sedimentary deposits now accumulating along the west coast of Europe. If now all these offshore formations were raised to open air, how could they be correlated?… All would be similar, however, in the fossils which they contain.

Some fossil species would be identical in all these formations and others would be closely allied. Making all due allowance for differences in species due to local differences in climate and other physical causes, it would still be plain that plants and animals so similar lived at the same period of time, and that the formations in which their remains were imbedded were contemporaneous in a broad way.

The presence of the bones of whales and other marine mammals would prove that the strata were laid after the appearance of mammals upon earth, and imbedded relics of man would give a still closer approximation to their age. In the same way we correlate the earlier geological formations.

GO ON TO THE NEXT PAGE.

13. According to the passage, each geological feature can serve as a site for a mineral vein EXCEPT:

A. porous and soluble rock.
B. fissure veins.
C. sandstone.
D. gold ores.

14. In the context of the passage, the word *lithologically* most nearly refers to:

A. composition and texture.
B. elevation.
C. geographical location.
D. fossil content.

15. The author suggests which of the following about geology?

A. The zone of cementation exists below the zone of solution.
B. Two categories of veins exist.
C. Fossils of fish bones prove that the strata were laid after the appearance of mammals.
D. Zinc deposits would most likely appear in the zone of cementation.

16. The author provides an explanation or example in the passage for each of the following EXCEPT:

A. Lower levels of veins may contain large amounts of silver.
B. The origin of igneous rock and lava.
C. The absolute age of strata can be determined.
D. The formation of fissure veins.

17. The author would agree with which of the following statements:

A. Gold from igneous rock is useless.
B. Mineral veins are the original source of the metals of veins.
C. Western Europe and Georgia share similar rock formations.
D. New Mexico and the Mississippi valley share similar metal deposits.

18. According to the passage, which of the following fossil findings would the author consider most unexpected?

A. Two different plant specimens in the same strata of earth from the same geographic region.
B. Two different plant specimens in two different strata of earth from different geographic regions.
C. Two similar plant specimens in two different strata of earth from the same geographic region.
D. Two similar plant specimens in two similar strata of earth from different geographic regions.

GO ON TO THE NEXT PAGE.

Passage IV (Questions 19 - 23)

Tracing the feeling back to its origin, it seems due to this: minds of the lower order can never see anything go wrong without experiencing a certain sense of resentment; and resentment, by its very nature, desires to vent itself upon some living and sentient creature, by preference a fellow human being.

When the child, running too fast, falls and hurts itself, it gets instantly angry. "Naughty ground to hurt baby!" says the nurse: "Baby hit it and hurt it." And baby promptly hits it back, with vicious little fist, feeling every desire to revenge itself. By-and-by, when baby grows older and learns that the ground can't feel to speak of, he wants to put the blame upon somebody else, in order to have an object to expend his rage upon. "You pushed me down!" he says to his playmate, and straightway proceeds to punch his playmate's head for it—not because he really believes the playmate did it, but because he feels he must have some outlet for his resentment. When once resentment is roused, it will expend its force on anything that turns up handy…

The mob, enraged at the death of Cæsar, meets Cinna the poet in the streets of Rome. "Your name, sir?" inquires the Third Citizen. "Truly, my name is Cinna," says the unsuspecting author. "Tear him to pieces!" cries the mob; "he's a conspirator!" "I am Cinna the poet," pleads the unhappy man; "I am not Cinna the conspirator!" But the mob does not heed such delicate distinctions at such a moment. "Tear him for his bad verses!" it cries impartially. "Tear him for his bad verses!"…

The fact is, the death is regarded as a misfortune, and somebody must be blamed for it. Heaven has provided scapegoats. The doctor and the hostile female members of the family are always there—laid on, as it were, for the express purpose…

In the Middle Ages, however, the pursuit of the scapegoat ran a vast deal further. When any great one died—a Black Prince or a Dauphin—it was always assumed on all hands that he must have been poisoned.

True, poisoning may then have been a trifle more frequent; certainly the means of detecting it were far less advanced… Still, people must often have died natural deaths even in the Middle Ages—though nobody believed it. All the world began to speculate that Jane Shore could have poisoned them. A little earlier, again, it was not the poisoner that was looked for, but his predecessor, the sorcerer. Whoever fell ill, somebody had bewitched him. Were the cattle diseased? Then search for the evil eye. Did the cows yield no milk? Some neighbor, doubtless, knew the reason only too well, and could be forced to confess it by liberal use of the thumb-screw and the ducking-stool. No misfortune was regarded as due to natural causes; for in their philosophy there were no such things as natural causes at all…

Our ancestors really believed there was always somebody to blame—man, witch, or spirit—if only you could find him; and though we ourselves have mostly got beyond that stage, yet the habit it engendered in our race remains ingrained in the nervous system, so that none but a few of the naturally highest and most civilized dispositions have really outgrown it… "Who fills the butcher's shops with large blue flies?" asked the poet of the Regency. He set it down to "the Corsican ogre."… There are just a few men here and there in the world who can see that when misfortunes come, circumstances, or nature, or (hardest of all) we ourselves have brought them. The common human instinct is still to get into a rage, and look round to discover whether there's any other fellow standing about unobserved, whose head we can safely undertake to punch for it.

 GO ON TO THE NEXT PAGE.

19. The main argument of the passage is that:

A. resentment goes further than vague verbal outbursts of temper.
B. the natural and instinctive desire of the human animal is to find a scapegoat.
C. whatever sort of misfortune falls upon people, they will always blame something.
D. we have ourselves to blame for misfortune.

20. According to the passage, the response of the crowd towards Cinna the poet:

A. Helps confirm that our ancestors believed there was always someone to blame.
B. Reveals the true unreasonable nature of people.
C. Embodies the universal impulse of humanity.
D. Supports the claim that resentment prefers to blame an innocent victim.

21. Which of the following scenarios would the author find most surprising?

A. A teenage girl stomping the sidewalk where she tripped.
B. A cab driver blaming his flat tire on the black bird that flew across his window.
C. A boy suspecting that his dead relative turned out the lights during a thunder storm.
D. A professor arguing with his wife, and kicking his dog for trying to follow him out of the house.

22. Which of the following statements, if true, would most *strengthen* the author's argument about scapegoats:

A. The Athenians kept a small collection of public scapegoats always in stock, waiting to be sacrificed at a moment's notice.
B. The Romans persecuted scapegoats without a fair trial.
C. The Byzantines forbade scapegoats from entering politics.
D. The Saracens punished public officers who habitually blamed others.

23. According to one chief of a village, "all deaths that occur in life are violent deaths, and are brought about by human or superhuman agency." Upon finding his brother dead on the ground, this chief would probably:

A. call for a physician to diagnose the probable cause of death.
B. call for an officer to hunt down the person responsible.
C. put in jail the person at the crime scene.
D. assign a witch-finder to disclose the evil spirit at work

———————————————————

GO ON TO THE NEXT PAGE.

Passage V (Questions 24 - 30)

By its influence the effects of calamity are spread so widely that they cease to be felt as calamity. The fact of death can not be set aside, but through insurance it need not appear as economic disaster, only as personal loss. Its essential nature is that of social cooperation and it furnishes some of the most effective of bonds which knit society together.

To all the interests of insurance, the lawlessness of war is wholly adverse and destructive. Insurance involves mutual trust and trust thrives under security of person and property. Insurance demands steadiness of purpose and continuity of law. In war, all laws are silent. War is the brutish, blind, denial of law, only admissible when all other honorable alternatives have been withdrawn--the last resort of "murdered, mangled liberty."

In its direct relation, war destroys those who to the underwriter represent the "best risks," the men most valuable to themselves and thus most valuable to the community. Those whom war leaves behind, to slip along the lines of least resistance into the city slums, are the people insurance rarely reaches. War confuses administration of insurance. Policies, in war time, can be written only on a sliding scale. This greatly increases the premium by reducing the final payments. Increase of rate of premium must decrease business. War means financial anarchy, inflated currency and depreciation of bonds. A currency which fluctuates demoralizes all business and war leaves no alternative.

The slogan "business as usual" in war time deceives nobody. If it did, nobody would gain by the deception. Enforced loans from the reserve fund of insurance companies to the state mean the depreciation of reserves. The substitution of unstable government bonds means robbery of the bond holders. The yielding to the state, by enforced "voluntary action," of reserves of savings banks and insurance companies represents a form of state robbery. This is now in practice on the continent of Europe. Such funds are probably never actually confiscated but held in abeyance until the close of the war. This is another form of the ever present "military necessity," which seizes men's property with little more compunction than it shows in seizing men's bodies. War conditions mean insecurity of investment. In war, all bonds are liable to become "scraps of paper," and no fund can be made safe. The insurance investments in Europe have been enormously depleted in worth, a reduction in market value estimated at 50 per cent.

Experts in insurance tell me that in wartime certain policies are written so as to be scaled down automatically when the holder goes under the colors. Some are invalid in time of war, and some have the clause of free travel greatly abridged... Companies generally refuse to pay under conditions not nominated under the bond, and in general, all policies are automatically reduced to level of war policies when war begins.

I am told that some American companies issue group policies as for any or all of a thousand men, these not subject to a physical examination.

In every regard, the business of insurance is naturally allied with the forces that make for peace... The same remark applies in some degree to every honorable or constructive business.

"Eternal vigilance is the price of liberty." The interests involved should put honest business on its guard. The insurance men could afford to maintain a thousand observers, men wise in business as well as in International Law, and in the manners and customs of the people of the world. A few dozen skillful politico-military detectives... These should watch the standing incentives to war. Such men should stand guard against the influences that work toward conflict. Those who work for peace should be not "firemen to be called in to put out the fire" already started through the negligence of business men...

GO ON TO THE NEXT PAGE.

24. The overall theme of the passage is that:

A. Economic stability is the groundwork for social protection.
B. Of the many forms of financial relation among men, none is more important than insurance.
C. The protection and social cooperation of insurance depends on economic stability.
D. Eternal vigilance prevents war and calamity.

25. Which of the following statements, if true, could explain very heavy war claims in a given country?

A. A large proportion of artisans and upper class did not participate in war.
B. Group policies began to subject members to physical examinations.
C. A large proportion of students and well-paid men were first to enlist.
D. A large proportion of uninsured men died in the war.

26. Which factors threaten the business of insurance?

    I.   increase of loans.
    II.   exhaustion of reserves.
    III.   the precarious nature of investment

A. I only
B. II only
C. I and III only
D. I, II, and III

27. The author probably views life insurance as:

A. essentially altruistic.
B. a necessary yet risky utility.
C. a selfish service.
D. surreptitious.

28. According to the passage, which of the following statements can be inferred about fire insurance?

A. All fire insurance contracts in foreign nations are held in abeyance until the close of war.
B. Based on a sliding scale, lower and upper class pay the same fire insurance premiums.
C. Fire insurance policies are scaled down automatically in the event of a fire.
D. Fire insurance policies are not as prone to the effects of war as those of life insurance.

29. Which statement about business during times of war reinforces the views of the author?

A. Many businesses feel unsafe about investing in bonds.
B. Businesses scale down during times of war.
C. Insurance companies create an economic environment that does not foster peace.
D. War slowly destroys business and economic welfare.

30. The passage suggests that the people who stand guard at all times for the security of business should be like:

A. firemen extinguishing a fire.
B. fireproof building material.
C. policemen investigating crimes.
D. a magnifying glass

———————————————————————

GO ON TO THE NEXT PAGE.

Passage VI (Questions 31 - 35)

Apparently no one qualified for the bounty on flax for, in 1661, provision was made for importing some flax seed from England. No price was fixed, in 1666, on "flax by reason of the uncertainty of the quality."

…It was also ordered that every tithable person should produce one pound of dressed hemp and one pound of dressed flax or two pounds of either annually. From that time on considerable hemp and flax were raised in Virginia, but most of the crop was used at home. Linen cloth was highly prized. There was also a demand for cordage made of hemp fibers for ships.

As already noted, the initial attempts of the colonists to grow the grains with which they had been accustomed in England came to naught. They were familiar with wheat, rye, barley and oats. To make satisfactory yields, these grains had to be broadcasted on well prepared seed beds. Newly cleared forests left the soil full of stumps and roots. The wooden plows of those days were useless on these newly cleared lands. Preparation of the soil, for tobacco or maize, could be accomplished with a hand hoe or shovel. These plants required space in which to develop their full growth. A tobacco plant could be set or a hill of corn planted wherever a little loose dirt could be found. Some English grains were seeded in the cleared land near Hampton and Newport News but these old fields, abandoned by the Indians, were also near to exhaustion. An "indifferent crop" was reported.

Hogs contributed more to the material welfare of the Jamestown Colony than historians have generally recognized. Hogs have many advantages over other breeds of livestock. They multiply much faster than any other domestic animal except poultry. They make faster gains and double the weight for the food consumed than do cattle, sheep or goats. When slaughtered, hogs dress out about 75 percent edible meat, as compared with 55 to 60 percent for cattle. When given wide open range in humid climates such as prevailed in the Tidewater, they do fairly well without other feed than what they can find for themselves.

In summer, at Jamestown, they obtained most of their living in the numerous fresh-water swamps. Tuckahoe, a flag-like swamp plant, with an enormous root system, was their favorite hot weather forage. The roots of tuckahoe, often as large as a man's arm, contain a crystalline acid that burns the mouth of a human being like fire. After a few trials, hogs seem to relish it. While tuckahoe is not a fattening feed, hogs eating it make satisfactory gains in weight.

Of all the domestic animals brought from England to Jamestown in the early days of the settlement, the most expensive to transport and the most useless after they arrived in Virginia were horses. The estimate of the number in the Colony in 1649 is 200. There was no purpose for them to serve. The fragile wooden plows of the seventeenth century were of no use among the stumps and roots in newly cleared forest lands. Horses were of no value for transportation as there were no roads through the forests or bridges over the rivers.

They were of little use as beasts of burden as there were few burdens to carry. A horse was no match for an able-bodied man on Indian trails through timbered country. As late as 1671, the Batts and Fallam expedition, consisting of five white men and seven Indians, who were the discoverers of New River, had horses for the white men when they left Petersburg. All of these animals were dead before they reached the mountains.

GO ON TO THE NEXT PAGE.

31. Which of the following describes the logical organization of the passage?

A. A main idea is presented, followed by several examples that support that idea.
B. Four main examples are presented, followed by the main argument.
C. Four main examples are presented with major arguments woven into them..
D. Four different examples are introduced to form an overall impression.

32. According to the passage, grains seeded in each of the following would most likely result in an indifferent crop EXCEPT:

A. spacious soil.
B. land prepared by Indians.
C. newly cleared forest.
D. any cleared land.

33. Suppose the government fixed the price of sweet potatoes at one hundred and fifty pounds sterling per one thousand pounds. Such a decision would most likely indicate:

A. Adequate land was cleared for farming potatoes.
B. A drop in price of commodities competing with sweet potatoes.
C. A rise in the number of sweet potato producers.
D. Very dependable growing conditions.

34. Each of the following statements would conflict with the author's understanding of commodities in Colonial America, EXCEPT:

A. Historians understood the utility of all livestock.
B. Food given to livestock was suitable for colonists.
C. Colonists struggled to grow oats.
D. Colonists elected to grow hemp and flax.

35. Suppose the colonists brought donkeys from England to Jamestown instead of horses. The most likely reaction the colonists would have to this animal would be:

A. Acceptance, because they would cost less than horses.
B. Relief, because donkeys could pull the wooden plows.
C. Disappointment, because there were few burdens to carry.
D. Frustration, because donkeys would die before reaching the mountains.

_____

GO ON TO THE NEXT PAGE.

Passage VII (Questions 36 - 40)

The Nirang is the urine of cow, ox, or she-goat, and the rubbing of it over the face and hands is the second thing a Parsee does after getting out of bed.

While the scholars of Europe are thus engaged in disinterring the ancient records of the religion of Zoroaster, it is of interest to learn what has become of that religion in those few settlements where it is still professed by small communities.

Though every religion is of real and vital interest in its earliest state only, yet its later development too, with all its misunderstandings, faults, and corruptions, offers many an instructive lesson to the thoughtful student of history.

Here is a religion, one of the most ancient of the world, once the state religion of the most powerful empire, driven away from its native soil, deprived of political influence, without even the prestige of a powerful or enlightened priesthood, and yet professed by a handful of exiles--men of wealth, intelligence, and moral worth in Western India--with an unhesitating fervor such as is seldom to be found in larger religious communities.

It is well worth the serious consideration of the philosopher and the divine to discover, if possible, the spell by which this apparently effete religion continues to command the attachment of the enlightened Parsis of India, and makes them turn a deaf ear to the allurements of the Brahmanic worship and the earnest appeals of Christian missionaries.

Far from being the teachers of the true doctrines and duties of their religion, the priests are generally the most bigoted and superstitious, and exercise much injurious influence over the women especially, who, until lately, received no education at all.

The priests have, however, now begun to feel their degraded position. Many of them, if they can do so, bring up their sons in any other profession but their own.

There are, perhaps, a dozen among the whole body of professional priests who lay claim to a knowledge of the Zend-Avesta: but the only respect in which they are superior to their brethren is, that they have learnt the meanings of the words of the books as they are taught, without knowing the language, either philosophically or grammatically.

The Reformers maintain that there is no authority whatever in the original books of Zurthosht for the observance of this unsanitary practice, but that it is altogether a later introduction.

The old adduce the authority of the works of some of the priests of former days, and say the practice ought to be observed. They quote one passage from the Zend-Avesta corroborative of their opinion, which their opponents deny as at all bearing upon the point.
The Reformers have found themselves strengthened by the intolerant bigotry and the weakness of the arguments of their opponents.

The Liberals have made considerable progress, but their work is as yet but half done, and they will never be able to carry out their religious and social reforms successfully, without first entering on a critical study of the Zend-Avesta, to which, as yet, they profess to appeal as the highest authority in matters of faith, law, and morality.

GO ON TO THE NEXT PAGE.

36. The priests who follow the Zend-Avesta best illustrate the author's point that:

A. Religion cannot teach the philosophical or grammatical aspects of language.
B. Superstition allows one to have influence over others.
C. Learning religion with knowledge of philosophy and grammar is respectable.
D. Language is not a prerequisite for knowledge.

37. Which of the following statements, if true, would most *strengthen* the argument of The Liberals?

A. Passages from the Zend-Avesta have been found in recent versions of the Zurthosht.
B. The Parsis of India have come to agreement on the authority of the Zend-Avesta.
C. The practice of rubbing Nirang on one's body has been found in the original books of Zurthosht.
D. The Reformers retract their accusations of bigotry and weakness.

38. The Oxford English Dictionary defines religion as "a pursuit or interest followed with devotion." If the author were to include this description in the passage, it would probably be used to:

A. illustrate the point that followers of a religion remain faithful despite eventual misunderstandings and corruption.
B. emphasize that the integrity and lessons of a religion dwindle over time.
C. explain the author's admiration for the Zoroaster religion.
D. support the point that followers of Zoroaster remain loyal to their faith.

39. The reference to Nirang shows primarily that:

A. There is disagreement among priests about Zoroastrian practices.
B. Priests who follow the Zend-Avesta are superstitious.
C. The author favors the views of The Reformers.
D. There is no authority whatever in the original books of Zurthosht.

40. According to the passage, The Reformers would disagree with each of the following ideas EXCEPT:

A. Unsanitary practices do not belong in their religion.
B. The books of Zurthosht are not the highest authority in matters of faith, law, and morality.
C. Knowing the philosophy of a culture is important to knowing its religion.
D. The Liberals have made progress, but are small-minded.

STOP.   IF YOU FINISH BEFORE TIME IS CALLED, CHECK YOUR WORK. YOU MAY GO BACK TO ANY QUESTION IN THIS TEST.

STOP.

SOLUTIONS AND EXPLANATIONS

MCAT Verbal Reasoning

WARM-UP PASSAGE

ANSWERS AND EXPLANATIONS

Warm-up Passage _____

1. The author's central thesis is that:

A. in wartime, an alternative to fighting battles exists. [True, but too broad.]
B. the pacific blockade is a kind of sport. [True, but too specific.]
C. coercion by maritime force is superior to open hostilities. [Coercion by maritime force may specify naval battles causing open hostilities, or blockades. This is too vague.]
D. blockades can be more effective than swift destruction. [Yes. The author argues that blockades are superior to fighting.]

2. The use of the pacific blockade would have what expected effect on a nation?
   - I. Dramatic increase in unemployment.
   - II. Extensive growth of the indigent population.
   - III. Starvation of animals.

A. I only [No. All three are expected to happen.]
B. III only [No. All three are expected to happen.]
C. I and II only [No. All three are expected to happen.]
D. I, II and III [All three are correct. Paragraph 2 explains that a blockade will sap the region of food and moral resources. "The interest largely depends on the duration of the blockade, and its duration on the victims' physical and moral resources…"]

3. The author suggests that the ultimate object of the blockade is to:

A. cause widespread starvation. [A tempting choice as the author explains this consequence in paragraph 2. But starvation is not the ultimate goal.]
B. propagate rebellion. [Correct. The author uses the example of the French cruisers to bring home the point that blockades are meant to cause the overthrow of a government. "French cruisers stopped the fishing-smacks and asked if their community had joined the Rebellion. When the answer was in the negative, they sank the vessel and confiscated the tackle, often accompanying the robbery of property with violence on the persons of the owners and abuse of their sovereign. To the wretched fishermen's protests, the French commanders replied: "If you want to be left alone, you have only to drive out your King."]
C. deplete physical and moral resources. [Another tempting choice as the author explains this consequence in paragraph 3. But rebellion is the ultimate goal.]
D. acquire control of a nation. [This is probably but not necessarily true. The attacking forces want to cause rebellion.]

Warm-up Passage

4. According to the passage, a nation can enact a blockade once it:

A. becomes a maritime power. [A tempting choice, but the author specifies that the blockading forces must first surpasses the resisting nation in force.]
B. declares war on another nation. [Incorrect.]
C. **surpasses the resisting nation in force. [Correct. "For it can only be employed as a measure of coercion by maritime Powers able to bring into action such vastly superior forces to those the resisting State can dispose of, that resistance is out of the question."]**
D. achieves a favorable economy. [No.]

5. A blockade would first cause the cessation of all maritime traffic, followed by what effect on the recipient nation?

A. Cessation of industry, followed by rising poverty. [Cessation of industry follows the suffering of the people.]
B. Rise in poverty, followed by cessation of industry. [Poverty makes sense, but the author specifically focuses on starvation first.]
C. Rise in disease, followed by cessation of industry. [Disease makes sense, but the author specifically focuses on starvation first.]
D. **Rise in starvation, followed by a cessation of industry. [Correct. "…he can see the victim going through the successive stages of misery--debility, languor, exhaustion—until the final point is reached; and as his scientific curiosity is gratified by the gradual manifestation of the various symptoms, so his moral sense is fortified by the struggle between a proud spirit and an empty stomach…"]**

6. Which of the following statements, if true, would most weaken the author's claim that blockade is not war, but a kind of sport?

A. Blockades affect the strongest side of the opposing nation first. [No.]
B. The assailant inevitably suffers losses. [This does not weaken the author's claim.]
C. **Maritime fleets enforcing the blockade engage in hostilities with the opposing nation. [Correct. The author states that the blockade avoids open hostilities. So answer choice C would strongly challenge this. "First, instead of the barbarous effusion of blood and swift destruction which open hostilities entail, the** pacific blockade achieves its ends by more refined and leisurely means…"]
D. Blockades cause swift destruction of opposing nations that are weak. [Incorrect.]

Verbal Test 1

Answers and Explanations

1. The author's major thesis is that:

A. Native Americans used cists for several key purposes. [Incorrect. Too general.]
B. The Navaho treated the dead in a remarkable manner. [Incorrect. Too specific.]
C. **The Navaho utilized cists in a number of ways that often overlapped in function. [Correct. This answer captures the proper level of focus of the passage.]**
D. The Navaho built cists for specific purposes. [Incorrect. Too vague.]

2. Which of the following assertions is NOT clearly supported by historical evidence provided by the passage author?

A. Water was seldom stored. [Incorrect. This is supported. "The storage of water was so seldom attempted, or perhaps so seldom necessary, that only one example of a reservoir was found."]
B. Some Navaho storage cists could not be differentiated from those of old pueblo. [Incorrect. This is supported. "Immense numbers of these storage cists are found in the canyon, some of them with masonry so roughly executed that it is difficult to discriminate between the old pueblo and the modern Navaho work."]
C. The Navaho respected their dead. [Incorrect. This is supported. "The number of burial cists in the canyon is remarkable; there are hundreds of them. Practically every ruin whose walls are still standing contains one or more, some have eight or ten. They are all of Navaho origin…"]
D. **Navaho storage cists were also used for habitation. [Correct. The author thinks this is probable, but does not provide evidence for it. "It is probable that many of the cliff outlooks themselves were used quite as much for temporary storage as for habitations during the farming season."]**

3. The author treats the idea of the antiquity of the Navaho ruins as:

A. difficult to access. [Incorrect. The burial cists are difficult to access, not the idea of antiquity.]
B. credible and sacred to the culture. [Incorrect. The author probably believes the ruins are credible and sacred, but never states this.]
C. **inseparable from the taboo of the dead. [Correct. "the Navaho taboo of their own dead has brought about the partial taboo of the cliff dwellers' remains which prevails, and which is an element that must be taken into account in any discussion of the antiquity of the ruins."]**
D. evidence for the use of cists as sites of temporary storage. [Incorrect.]

4. Which of the following inferences is justified by information in the passage?

A. **The Navaho believed in some form of afterlife. [Correct. The Navaho buried their dead in coves high above the ground in cliffs. This suggests that they made a connection between burial location, and some special meaning for those they buried.]**
B. Storage and habitation were a priority for the Navaho. [Incorrect. Evidence in the passage makes this obvious.]
C. A similar people, the old pueblo, came before the Navaho. [Incorrect. Evidence in the passage makes this obvious.]
D. Some catastrophic event struck the Navaho people. [Incorrect. The fact that they had hundreds of burial cists does not necessarily suggest that many people died from a catastrophe.]

5. The author of the passage seems to hold the opinion that:

A. **The Navaho possessed large containers for water storage. [Correct. "…a supply of water must have been kept in them, and where this requirement was common… some receptacle other than jars of pottery would be provided."]**
B. Members of the Navaho were tall and fit. [A tempting answer, but incorrect. Yes, the author believes the Navaho are fit, but makes no mention of height.]
C. The Navaho were attacked often by invaders. [Incorrect.]
D. Many civilizations used storage cists. [Incorrect. The author does not discuss cists of many civilizations]

Answers and Explanations

6. Which of the following statements is inconsistent with information in the passage?

A. Chaldea contained famous places of holiness. [Incorrect. This is supported. "…Chaldea… was the cradle of nations which afterwards grew to greatness… was regarded as a place of peculiar holiness."]
B. European explorers visited Erech. [Incorrect. This is supported.]
C. The dead were confiscated from Assyrian cities. [Correct. The author remarks that perhaps the Assyrians themselves removed their own dead.]
D. A very large site of buried citizens is sometimes referred to as a Necropolis. [Incorrect. This is supported. "…around it gradually formed an immense "city of the dead" or Necropolis."]

7. Which of the following inferences is justified by information in the passage?

A. Chaldean cities became a Necropolis. [Incorrect. This is clearly stated, and is not an inference.]
B. The Egyptians buried their dead in pots. [Incorrect. There is no suggestion of this.]
C. Temples of Babylonia suffered considerable damage. [Incorrect. There is not enough evidence to infer that damage caused the "shapeless masses."]
D. Some regions of Chaldea are submerged under swamps in May. [Correct. "…Warka and a few other mounds are raised on a slightly elevated tract of the desert, above the level of the yearly inundations, and accessible only from November to March…"]

8. The author of the passage probably most strongly supports:

A. proper burial of the dead. [Incorrect. The author never provides an opinion on this.]
B. logical arguments supported by evidence. [Correct. The author values evidence for support. "The latter conjecture, though not entirely devoid of foundation, as we shall see, is unsupported by any positive facts, and therefore was never seriously discussed."]
C. places of holiness. [Incorrect. The author never provides an opinion on this.]
D. written history. [Incorrect. The author puts more faith in physical evidence. "To this loving veneration for the dead history owes half its discoveries; indeed we should have almost no reliable information at all on the very oldest races, who lived before the invention of writing, were it not for their tombs and the things we find in them."]

9. If information in the passage is accurate, which of the following would one LEAST expect to find in ancient Assyria?

A. Empty tombs. [Incorrect. Empty tombs are expected. "It is a curious fact that in Assyria the ruins speak to us only of the living, and that of the dead there are no traces whatever."]
B. Greatly decorated final resting places that are intricately designed. [Incorrect. This would be expected. "Yet it is well known that all nations have bestowed as much care on the interment of their dead and the adornment of their last resting-place as on the construction of their dwellings…]
C. Temples of shapeless masses. [Correct. The author indicates that all artistic evidence disappeared from Babylonian temples, and that this is contrary to Assyria.]
D. Designated locations of buried precious metals. [Incorrect. The passage never makes any reference to treasure, so we cannot say for certain whether or not treasure had specific locations.]

10. The author apparently believes that burial of the dead in great numbers in a single region is:

A. odd, especially if continued to present day. [Correct. The example of Chaldea is a prime example. "Strangely enough, some portions of it even now are held sacred in the same sense."]
B. not surprising if done using sepulchers. [Incorrect.]
C. correlated with the degree of holiness of an ancient city. [Incorrect. The author does not make this correlation.]
D. expected in civilizations high in culture. [Incorrect. There is no connection made between the number of dead buried in a location and the degree of culture.]

11. Several cities and civilizations cited in the passage revealed unexpected findings EXCEPT for:

A. modern Turkey. [Correct. "the sepulchers which are found in such numbers in some mounds down to a certain depth, belong, as is shown by their very position, to later races, mostly even to the modern Turks and Arabs."]
B. Warka. [Incorrect. Loftus was very surprised by his discoveries in Warka.]
C. Assyria. [Incorrect. "It is a curious fact that in Assyria the ruins speak to us only of the living, and that of the dead there are no traces whatever."]
D. Chaldea. [Incorrect. "Strangely enough, some portions of it even now are held sacred in the same sense."]

12. It can most justifiably be said that the main purpose of the passage is:

A. **to describe defensible theories of timber splits and shakes. [Correct. The author describes shakes and splits in timber.]**
B. to clarify the principles of freezing wood. [Incorrect. Too narrow. The passage goes beyond trying to explain the effects of freezing wood.]
C. to outline an analysis of tree damage. [Incorrect. Too broad. The focus is on splits and shakes, not all forms of tree damage.]
D. to evaluate mechanisms of frost damage. [Incorrect. Too broad. The focus is on timber.]

13. According to the passage, simple heart shake causes primarily which of the following forms of damage?

A. **One cleft across the pith. [Correct. "When it consists of a single cleft extending across the pith it is termed simple heart shake."]**
B. A hollow hole with radial clefts. [Incorrect. This describes typical heart shake.]
C. Several radial clefts. [Incorrect. This describes star shake.]
D. A cleft across one or two boards of spiral grained timber. [Incorrect. "Shake of this character in straight-grained trees affects only one or two central boards when cut into lumber, but in spiral-grained timber the damage is much greater."]

14. The author of the passage would be most likely to agree with which of the following ideas?

A. Radial splits extend inward and usually near the middle trunk. [Incorrect. Radial splits usually affect the base.]
B. Without cold temperatures, splits do not occur. [Incorrect. Mechanical stress from wind can be sufficient to cause splits.]
C. **The chemical nature of wood changes over time. [Correct. "It usually results from a shrinkage of the heartwood due probably to chemical changes in the wood."]**
D. Splits are more common than shakes. [Incorrect. The passage does not offer support for this statement.]

15. Suppose splits occurred on an old tree during a day of no wind. Busse would support which of the following statements as the most likely explanation?

A. The temperature rose above 14°F. [Incorrect. This would not explain how splits occurred on a windless day.]
B. **The frost alone produced enough tension to open old frost splits. [Correct. Busse attributes splits to frost and wind. In the absence of wind, frost is the main culprit.]**
C. Wet sites produced condensation inside the cell walls of the tree. [Incorrect. The passage does not offer a connection between wet sites and water in cell walls.]
D. Freezing forced out water from the cell walls. [Incorrect. This is Hartig's theory.]

16. On the basis of the passage, lighter-colored clefts in a converted hardwood that maintains its size over time is best described as:

A. Radial splits. [Incorrect.]
B. Star shake. [Incorrect.]
C. **Seasoning cracks. [Correct. "…clefts due to heart shake may be distinguished from seasoning cracks by the darker color of the exposed surfaces. Such clefts, however, tend to open up more and more as the timber seasons."]**
D. Heart shake. [Incorrect. Heart shake is darker colored and widens over time. "…clefts due to heart shake may be distinguished from seasoning cracks by the darker color of the exposed surfaces. Such clefts, however, tend to open up more and more as the timber seasons."]

17. Which of the following statements, if true, would most directly challenge the mechanical theory of radial splits?

A. Freezing forces water into cell walls. [Incorrect. The mechanical theory is by Busse. This would directly challenge the theory by Hartig.]
B. **Tension is always in excess of pressure. [Correct. This would directly attack the theory by Busse which states that "…only where the pressure is in excess of the tension, i.e., between the roots, can a separation of the fiber result."]**
C. Difference in temperature between inner and outer layers is insufficient to set up strains. [Incorrect. This would weaken the second, unidentified theory on splits. It would not impact the theory by Busse.]
D. Most splits take place after sunrise. [Incorrect. This is a tempting answer, but not the best one. Splitting after sunrise is not the greatest challenge to Busse's theory.]

18. Elsewhere, the author of the passage states that ring shake results from the concentric as well as radial shrinkage of heartwood. Ring shake may occur in connection with what other form of damage?

A. Frost splits. [Incorrect.]
B. Radial splits. [Incorrect.]
C. Log shake. [Incorrect. The passage never mentions log shake.]
D. **Heart shake. [Correct. heart shake occurs due to shrinkage of the heartwood, exhibiting radial clefts. Radial shrinkage is a component of ring shake as indicated in the question.]**

19. According to the passage, a Particular Baptist would agree with each of the following tenets EXCEPT for:

A. justification. [Incorrect. "They believe in eternal election, free justification, ultimate glorification..."]
B. being particular. [Incorrect. They are very particular about their beliefs.]
C. open communion. [Correct. The General Baptists believe in open communion.]
D. baptism. [Incorrect. They believe in baptism.]

20. Suppose that the Particular Baptist Chapel were moved further away from the street. The most likely result of this action would be that:

A. Services would be held earlier in the mornings. [Incorrect.]
B. Calvinist membership would decrease. [Incorrect. The passage suggests membership would increase due to less noise.]
C. Fewer children would attend church. [Incorrect. The noise level would decrease.]
D. Membership would increase. [Correct. The passage suggests membership would increase due to less noise.]

21. Which of the following findings, if true, would suggest that the author's concern about unpleasant experiences is exaggerated?

A. The congregations are encouraged by elevated volumes. [Correct. If the congregations are encouraged by loud volumes, then the lengthy hymns and lively street sounds that the author complains about would not bother the congregations.]
B. People living in the Vauxhall-road district stop attending church. [Incorrect. This would support the author's observations that the loud streets and annoying hymns are indeed bothersome.]
C. Baptists convert to a different religion en masse. [Incorrect. This would not challenge the author's concern, and may be grounds to support it.]
D. Members of the Baptist Chapel ceased singing hymns in church. [Incorrect. This would not challenge the author's concern, and may be grounds to support it.]

22. On the basis of information in the passage, one would generally expect the members of Vauxhall-road Particular Baptist Chapel to be:

A. pious. [Incorrect.]
B. frugal. [Not the best answer. Frugal means economical, or avoiding waste. The author focuses on the chapel's lack of decoration, it's plain appearance.]
C. austere. [Correct. The chapel is very plain and simple, with nothing ornamental. Thus, it is austere, which reflects the taste of its members.]
D. quiet. [Incorrect. The chapel is described as appearing quiet, which does not necessarily mean the people are quiet.]

23. The example of the General Baptists is most relevant to the author's assertion that particular people in a religion:

A. **risk going too far to the detriment of its own members. [Correct. The author suggests that the rigid mandate for all members to become baptized may result in "a simple question of dryness."]**
B. miss opportunities to challenge their own thinking. [Incorrect. The author never mentioned this.]
C. trap themselves by becoming too rigid. [A tempting answer, but not the best. The author talks about the empty pail of baptism.]
D. are actually more particular than members of the Particular Baptists. [Incorrect.]

24. The author would question which of the following statements:

A. Calvinists are just as strict as Baptists. [Incorrect. The author likens Particular Baptists to Calvinists and sees them as similar.]
B. Unpopular people might be very particular. [Incorrect. The author would agree.]
C. **A handful of concepts involve particularity. [Correct. The author believes hundreds of things involve particularity. "Singularity, eccentricity, speciality, isolation, oddity, and hundreds of other things which might be mentioned, all involve particularity."]**
D. The various ways in which people decorate a building reflect more their tastes than their judgments. [Incorrect. The author would agree. "This is not intended as a reflection upon the occupants, but is done as a simple matter of taste."]

25. The assertion that tobacco has been cultivated in Mexico "from time immemorial" is:

A. contradicted by the assertion that the Spaniards introduced the plant to Mexico. [Incorrect. The author does not make this assertion.]
B. possibly true but not supported by examples or evidence. [Incorrect.]
C. **true, given the findings of explorers. [Correct. "Francisco Lopez de Gomara, who was chaplain to Cortez, when he made conquest of Mexico, in 1519, alludes to the plant…"]**
D. supported by objective data in the passage. [Incorrect.]

26. One can justifiably infer from the author's comments about tobacco that there exists:

A. **various kinds of plant, each with a distinct taste. [Correct. The final paragraph about the Yara makes this case.]**
B. dozens of kinds of plants. [Incorrect. While probably true, the author mentions fewer than ten.]
C. generations of crops of superior quality. [Incorrect. Second and third generation crops have inferior quality.]
D. wealthy merchants in the business of selling tobacco products. [Incorrect. The author never mentions merchants.]

27. Which of the following statements captures the sentiments of the author the LEAST?

A. The earliest use of tobacco was in the form of cigars. [Incorrect. The author would agree. "The smoking of tobacco in the form of cigars is doubtless the most general as well as the most ancient mode of its use."]
B. Without a doubt the Yara has an unnatural taste. [Incorrect. The author would agree. "." It can, doubtless, be said with truth concerning the Yara cigar, that… the taste for them is not natural…"]
C. People tend to appreciate one taste to the point of disliking other tastes. [Incorrect. The author makes this point in the Yara example.]
D. **Tobacco was highly valued, but not ubiquitously used among Native Americans. [Correct. The author believes that the smoking of the peace pipe was the most highly valued and <u>universal</u> custom among Native Americans.]**

28. The author would most likely disagree with which of the following statements about tobacco:

A. Natives of Central America used tobacco in the form of cigars. [Incorrect. The author would agree. "The smoking of tobacco in the form of cigars is doubtless the most general as well as the most ancient mode of its use. When Columbus landed in Hispaniola, the sailors saw the natives smoking the leaves of a plant…"]

B. In general, tobacco products have a pleasing flavor. [Correct. The author would not fully agree. The final paragraph about the Yara tasting bitter to most people makes this case.]

C. Cigars are made by using a binder, and truncating one end. [Incorrect. The author would agree. "divested of the stem and wound about with a binder, and enveloped in a portion of the leaf known by the name of wrapper—acute at one end and truncated at the other…"]

D. Overall, tobacco products from Manilla are as high in quality as those from Havana, and even London. [Incorrect. The author does not provide enough clues to indicate a preference.]

29. Which of the following examples in the passage regarding various uses of tobacco demonstrates irony?

A. The predilection of Londoners to smoke the Yara. [Incorrect. This is not ironic.]

B. The post-dinner ceremonies of king Montezuma. [Incorrect. This is not ironic.]

C. The burial rituals of Native Americans. [Correct. The author indicates that Native Americans were buried with a peace pipe and weapons of war such as the tomahawk. Their stark contrast creates the irony.]

D. The discoveries made by Columbus and Lopez de Gomara. [Incorrect. These are not ironic.]

30. For which of the following conclusions does the passage offer the most support?

A. Switzerland has too few restaurants. [Incorrect. "In most of the big towns the hotels have restaurants attached to them… There is in every little mountain-hotel a restaurant…"]
B. Colder climates favor fish as the main cuisine. [Incorrect. "Farther and farther south, as the climate becomes hotter, the meat becomes less and less the food of the people, various dishes of paste and fish taking its place …"]
C. Italian cuisine tastes better than that of all other nations. [Incorrect. This is never implied.]
D. The poor tend to misuse ingredients. [Correct. "Garlic is an excellent seasoning in its proper place and quantity, and the upper classes of the Spaniards have their meat lightly rubbed with it before being cooked, but the lower classes use it in the cooking to an intolerable extent."]

31. Which cuisine suffers from the greatest amount of undeserved criticism?

A. Spanish. [Incorrect.]
B. Austrian. [Incorrect.]
C. Swiss. [Incorrect.]
D. Italian. [Correct. "There is no cookery in Europe so often maligned without cause as that of Italy."]

32. Which of the following decisions based on Italian cuisine, if true, would best serve as an example for the candid Frenchman if he were living in Italy?

A. Despite the very oily taste of Italian cuisine, the contributions of Sorrento walnuts to French cuisine should be recognized. [Correct. The candid Frenchman failed to recognize Spain's contribution to French cuisine after being dissatisfied with its taste. This parallels that mistake, and corrects it.]
B. Despite the rumors that Italian cuisine is too oily, the contributions of Sorrento walnuts to French cuisine should be recognized. [Incorrect. This answer does not parallel the example of the candid Frenchman, because the Frenchman actually tasted Spain's cuisine.]
C. Despite the very oily taste of Italian cuisine, the contributions of Sorrento walnuts to Spanish cuisine should be recognized. [Incorrect. This answer does not parallel the example of the candid Frenchman, because the Frenchman ignored contributions to his own national cuisine.]
D. Despite the rumors that Italian cuisine is too oily, the contributions of Sorrento walnuts to Spanish cuisine should be recognized. [Incorrect. This answer does not parallel the example of the candid Frenchman, because the Frenchman actually tasted Spain's cuisine, and because the Frenchman ignored contributions to his own national cuisine.]

33. Assume that a Frenchman gave a favorable critique of the cuisine in Switzerland. The author would most likely find this critique:

A. somewhat surprising since the French are the most critical of cuisine from other nations. [Incorrect. The cuisine in Switzerland is as good as that of the French, so the author would not be surprised.]

B. probable, given the quality of à la carte dinners in big towns. [Correct. "In most of the big towns the hotels have restaurants attached to them, and in some of these a dinner ordered à la carte is just as well cooked as in a good French restaurant, and served as well…" French cooking was quite prevalent in Switzerland.]

C. remarkable, given the Frenchman's failure to realize Spain's contributions to French cuisine. [Incorrect. The cuisine in Switzerland is as good as that of the French, so the author would not be surprised.]

D. very surprising because Switzerland is a country of hotels and not of restaurants. [Incorrect. The cuisine in Switzerland is as good as that of the French, so the author would not be surprised.]

34. Suppose that the author could decide where to eat a dinner containing garlic and oil. Where would the author prefer to eat this meal?

A. Austria [Incorrect. Viennese cuisine is really French cuisine, except for the drink.]

B. Spain. [Incorrect. The author finds Spanish oil to be unrefined and unpleasant.]

C. Italy. [Correct. "whereas very little oil is used except at Genoa, where oil, and very good oil as a rule, takes the place of butter, and no more garlic than is necessary to give a slight flavor to the dishes in which it plays a part. An Italian cook fries better than one of any other nationality."]

D. Switzerland. [Incorrect.]

35. The author is primarily concerned with demonstrating that:

A. Morality serves the foundation for many cultures. [Incorrect.]
B. Religion is a complex entity that cannot be simplified. [Correct. The author explains in paragraph four that religions, like governments, cannot be agreed upon by all races.]
C. Myths, like religions, are unpredictable. [Incorrect.]
D. Mythologies from different cultures share common themes. [Incorrect.]

36. The author describes women as representing each of the following EXCEPT:

A. goodness. [Correct. The author never likens women to goodness in the passage.]
B. the invisible. [Incorrect. "These two women were perfectly beautiful, but invisible to the eyes of mortals."]
C. the mother of all mankind. [Incorrect. "…and by her begat the race of man."]
D. daylight. [Incorrect. "When the Woman of Light was at work, it was daytime."]

37. The author would most likely agree with which of the following about religion?

A. The source of all religion is self sacrifice.[Incorrect]
B. Religion and morality share a common purpose. [Incorrect]
C. The female element plays a central theme in religions. [Correct. The author offers examples of women playing a prominent role in religion in the first and second paragraphs.]
D. Animism lies at the heart of religion. [Incorrect.]

38. Which of the following, if true, would most weaken the author's argument?

A. Man has a basic desire for unlimited power. [Incorrect.]
B. Historical documents disprove the cultural imperative. [Incorrect.]
C. Archeologists discover religious texts describing mythological animals giving birth to all of mankind. [Incorrect.]
D. The basis of morality is hedonism. [Correct. Hedonism is the pursuit of pleasure as a matter of ethical principle, which is the opposite of self-sacrifice. This is in direct conflict with the author's claim that self-sacrifice is the basis for morality.]

39. The author states that "the brash wood of ancient date cannot be grafted on the green stem." The most likely purpose of this reference is to show that:

A. Old ideas cannot be imposed on younger generations. [Correct.]
B. Moral thought and religious life are a work-in-progress. [Incorrect.]
C. Many citizens do not desire a moral code. [Incorrect.]
D. Morality can undermine religion. [Incorrect.]

40. The word "heathendoms" most clearly represents:

A. Martyrs. [Incorrect.]
B. Philosophers. [Incorrect. The word refers to an independent approach to religion and morality.]
C. Agnostics. [Correct. A heathen is an irreligious, uncultured, or uncivilized person. In the context of the passage, heathendoms represents a throwing away of mainstream morality.]
D. Renegades. [Incorrect. This is too extreme.]

VERBAL TEST 2

ANSWERS AND EXPLANATIONS

1. The passage implies that a man who does not sing as he paints with a blue stick probably:

A. **does not believe that Tira´wahut can help him. [Correct. The last sentence reveals that man sings to powers because those powers help him. "The hills help man, so we sing to them." Blue is the color of the sky, the dwelling place of Tira´wahut. So if he does not believe the hills can help, he will not sing to them.]**
B. believes Toharu can help him instead. [Incorrect.]
C. does so out of respect for the sky. [Incorrect. This answer is making an assumption.]
D. is appealing to the lesser power of Silence. [There is no mention of a lesser power of Silence.]

2. According to the passage, each of the following lesser powers come down to help mankind EXCEPT:

A. Brown Eagle. [Incorrect. The passage indicates that this lesser power resides in the sky, which implies that it must take a path down to man in order to help man. "These lesser powers dwell in the great circle of the sky. One is North Star; another is Brown Eagle."]
B. Sun. [Incorrect. The passage indicates that this lesser power resides in the sky, which implies that it must take a path down to man in order to help man. "The Sun is one of these powers. It comes from the mighty power above"]
C. North Star. [Incorrect. The passage indicates that this lesser power resides in the sky, which implies that it must take a path down to man in order to help man. "These lesser powers dwell in the great circle of the sky. One is North Star; another is Brown Eagle."]
D. **Winds. [Correct. Winds do not need to come down from the sky because they are always near man. "They stand at the four points, and guard the four paths down which the lesser powers come when they help mankind. The Winds are always near us, by day and by night."]**

3. Suppose that the Pawnee believed that the ox represents the power which brings forth fighting strength, and that this power comes from the night. In the Hako, fighting power would most likely be represented by:

A. the Ox with an Owl painted on it. [Incorrect. The night does not come from the Owl, so the Owl would not be painted on the Ox.]
B. **the Ox painted with black. [Correct. As indicated in the passage, the power that is being invoked is painted with the power from which it comes. "The power which dwells in the earth, which enables it to give life to all growing things, comes from above. Therefore, in the Hako, the Pawnee ceremony, the ear of corn is painted with blue." In this hypothetical example, the ox comes from the night, which is black. Note that the ox does not come from the Owl. The Owl is the chief of the night.]**
C. the Owl painted with blue. [Incorrect.]
D. the Owl with an Ox painted on it. [Incorrect.]

4. According to the passage, the Pawnee would interpret the flame from a burning stick to be:

A. Sun speaking, since fire comes from the Sun. [Incorrect. The passage does not state that fire comes from the Sun.]
B. Mother Earth speaking, since all life comes from her. [Incorrect. This is an abstraction.]
C. Wood speaking, in answer to man's prayer. [Incorrect. The flame is the "word of the fire."]
D. **Fire speaking, with permission from Toharu. [Correct. "Fire… comes direct from the power granted Toharu… in answer to man's prayer as he rubs the sticks. When the flame leaps from the glowing wood, it is the word of the fire."]**

5. Suppose that Water was the first of the lesser powers to come near man. How would this impact man's call for aid?

A. **Man would make sure to live by a body of water. [Correct. Since Water would be the first of the lesser powers, man would call on it first. Just as the Winds always surrounded man and offered protection, man would want to stay within close range to Water to receive its protection.]**
B. Water would become the source of all lesser powers. [Incorrect. The Winds would be the first of the lesser powers, not the source of lesser powers. Tira'wa-tius, the Mighty Power, is the source of all lesser powers.]
C. Man would still call to the Winds first, since they are always near him. [Incorrect. Man calls on the first of the lesser powers, which in this example would be Water.]
D. Man could not call for aid because the Winds would be a lesser power. [Incorrect. Man could still call on the Winds for aid, but man would call on Water first since it is the first of the lesser powers.]

6. According to the author, what is the main factor that regulated the economy in the twentieth century?

A. Prices of imports from India. [Incorrect. Too narrow.]
B. Manufacturing in Russia, India, and Germany. [This is not the main factor.]
C. Cheap labor beyond the shores of England. [Incorrect. This is not the main factor.]
D. Colonies competing with England in their production of manufactured goods. [Correct. The author considers England to be the major colonizer, and discusses other national economies in comparison to English manufacturing.]

7. According to the passage, the business exploits of England merchants in India:

A. Suffered from a clash of cultures. [Correct. Indian weavers—artists and experts in their own craft—could not inure themselves to factory life... merchants had to adapt themselves to new conditions, now fully mastered, before British India could become the menacing rival of the Mother-land..."]
B. Struggled to understand the needs of workers in India. [The passage never indicates that the British made any attempt at understanding the needs of workers in India.]
C. Lost profit from broken machinery. [Not the best answer.]
D. Succeeded initially, but then succumbed to the failures of machinery and climate. [Incorrect. "At first a series of experiments ended in failure."]

8. With which of the following opinions would the author most likely *disagree*?

A. India is a country that should manufacture goods. [Incorrect. The author would agree with this. "And why should India not manufacture? What should be the hindrance?"]
B. Countries with cheap labor are limited by capital. [Correct. The author would not agree. "Capital?—But capital goes wherever there are men, poor enough to be exploited." Thus, capital is not considered to be a limiting factor.]
C. Laborers in industrialized nations are as skilled as workers in less developed countries. [Incorrect. The author would agree with this. "Are, then, Hindu workmen inferior to the hundreds of thousands of boys and girls, not eighteen years old, at present working in the English textile factories?"]
D. Business practices of English colonization evolved into a more exploitative power. [Incorrect. The author would agree with this. "...English merchants and capitalists conceived the very simple idea that it would be more expedient to exploit the natives of India by making cotton-cloth in India itself, than to import from twenty to twenty-four million pounds' worth of goods..."]

9. The example of Germany serves primarily to:

A. Explain the natural progression of industrious nations becoming economically independent. [Not necessarily true. The author does not say that all industrious nations will become economically independent.]
B. Highlight the inferior manufacturing of France and England. [Incorrect.]
C. Emphasize the growing competition faced by English manufacturing. [Incorrect.]
D. Give proof against the specialization of national industry. [Correct. Germany never suffered from exploitation by England precisely because it manufactured a broad spectrum of goods, unlike India which was a source of primarily raw textiles as indicated in the passage. English merchants exploited countries like India that focused on raw material exports.]

10. Suppose that a once-agricultural country such as Brazil evolved to become a manufacturing power of cotton. The author would most likely find this news to be:

A. a notable exception. [Incorrect.]
B. not surprising. [Correct. The author mentions countries like Russia and Poland which rose to manufacturing prominence in their respective industries.]
C. expected. [Incorrect. The author does not indicate any expectation that an agricultural country is to become a manufacturing power, but would not be surprised if one did.]
D. not possible given the theory of colonization. [Incorrect.]

11. Suppose that a tax on imported Russian goods into England were abolished. The most likely outcome of this action would be:

A. Sales of British goods in Russia would increase. [Incorrect.]
B. Sales of Russian goods in Russia would increase. [Incorrect.]
C. Sales of British goods in England would decrease. [Correct. "English capitalists, accompanied by engineers and foremen of their own nationalities, have introduced in Russia and in Poland manufactories whose goods compete in excellence with the best from England." Therefore, a drop in price of a Russian product, given its equal quality, would make Russian products more attractive to customers.]
D. No change due to the inferior quality of Russian goods. [Incorrect. The passage indicates that Russian goods were of excellent quality.]

12. Which of the following events, references, or ideas does not appear in the passage?

A. An astrological figure. [Incorrect. "But the Immortal was not wounded; on the other hand, his celestial dog jumped at Ch'an-yü and bit her neck…"]

B. A Roman general. [Incorrect. "The former was the chief superintendent of supplies for the armies of the tyrant emperor Chou, the Nero of China." Nero was a Roman emperor.]

C. A magical boy. [Correct. There is not reference to a boy in the passage.]

D. A military retreat. [Incorrect. "As a result of the fighting that ensued, Chiu-kung was beaten, and retreated in confusion…"]

13. The passage suggests that Têng Chiu-kung most likely felt:

A. proud of Ch'an-yü.

B. betrayed by T'u Hsing-sun. [Correct. T'u Hsing-sun was the magical healer of Têng Chiu-kung. Têng Chiu-kung offered his duaghter's hand in marriage to T'u Hsing-sun if he would win a pivotal battle for him in. Instead, Chiang Tzǔ-ya attacked and defeated Têng Chiu-kung to obtain his daughter, whom he handed over to T'u Hsing-sun. Têng Chiu-kung must have thus suspected that Chiang Tzǔ-ya and T'u Hsing-sun had communicated.]

C. cautious about Chü Liu-sun. [Incorrect. The passage never indicates or suggests that Têng Chiu-kung held an opinion of Chü Liu-sun.]

D. approval of Têng Hsiu. [Incorrect. While the passage does reveal Têng Hsiu to be the son of Têng Chiu-kung, it does not reveal how Têng Chiu-kung feels about his son.]

14. Conflict between each of the following pairs is depicted in the passage EXCEPT between:

A. the Chou Dynasty and Yin Dynasty. [Incorrect. Members of these dynasties fought against each other.]

B. the Yellow Flying Tiger and the Blower. [Incorrect. "…the combat continued until the Blower was wounded in the shoulder by No-cha, of the army of Chou, and pierced in the stomach with a spear by Huang Fei-hu, Yellow Flying Tiger…"]

C. the Blue Dragon and the Chou Dynasty. [Incorrect. Têng Chiu-kung, the Blue Dragon, fought against No-Cha of the Chou Dynasty. "There, in standing up to No-cha and Huang Fei-hu, he had his left arm broken by the former's magic bracelet…"]

D. the Snorter and the Blue Dragon. [Correct. The Snorter fought against the Blower, but not against Têng Chiu-kung, the Blue Dragon.]

15. According to the passage, Têng Chiu-kung fought on the side of:

A. the Yin Dynasty. [Incorrect. Têng Chiu-kung fought for both the Yin and Chou Dynasties at different times.]

B. the Chou Dynasty. [Incorrect. Têng Chiu-kung fought for both the Yin and Chou Dynasties at different times.]

C. both the Yin and Chou Dynasties. [Correct. Têng Chiu-kung was a member of the Yin Dynasty. After his daughter married into the Chou Dynasty, Têng Chiu-kung fought for the Chou. "In the ensuing battles he fought valiantly on the side of his former enemy, and killed many famous warriors…"]

D. neither the Yin nor Chou Dynasties. [Incorrect.]

16. The passage depicts the columns of light of the Snorter, and the yellow gas of the Blower. This is a reflection of:

A. an author attempting to add a sense of immortality to venerated Chinese military generals. [Incorrect. The writer of this passage did not invent these characters. They derive from Chinese folklore.]

B. factual military leaders who served in the ancient Chinese army. [Incorrect. This passage speaks of Chinese folklore.]

C. an author staying true to Chinese folklore. [Correct. The Snorter and the Blower depict ancient Chinese folklore.]

D. ancient Chinese fiction. [Not the best answer. In the context of Chinese mythology, supernatural characters are considered folklore, not fiction.]

17. Which of the following discoveries, if true, would most *weaken* the author's argument?

A. An anarchist Commune that feeds and clothes all of its members. [Incorrect. The author expects this. "… the anarchist Commune… understands that while it produces all that is necessary to material life, it must also strive to satisfy all manifestations of the human mind."]

B. A Communist society in which each member owns a scientific instrument. [Correct. The author's main argument against Communist society is that it fails to meet the artistic and leisure needs of its people. The author considers a scientific instrument to be an item of leisure, and would thus not expect everyone to own one "…beautiful pictures, optical instruments, luxurious furniture…"]

C. A social revolution that guarantees daily bread for all. [Incorrect.]

D. A free society that engages in a revolution and becomes Communist. [There is no mention of free societies.]

18. Each of the following statements is supported by the passage EXCEPT:

A. Tastes vary, but artistic needs exist in all. [Incorrect. The author would agree. "As soon as his material wants are satisfied, other needs, which, generally speaking, may be described as of an artistic character, will thrust themselves forward."]

B. Some citizens like statues, some like pictures. [This is nearly a direct quote. "Some like statues, some like pictures."]

C. Clothing all members is sufficient for a society to exist. [Correct. The main argument of the author is that meeting the basic needs of a society is not enough. A society must meet the higher needs of its citizens.]

D. The exploitation of labor is not uncommon. [Incorrect. The author believes this. "If we wish for a Social Revolution… to transform this execrable society, in which we can every day see capable workmen dangling their arms for want of an employer who will exploit them…"]

19. The passage addresses an important relationship between:

A. Leisure and the success of the social revolution. [Not the best answer. The immediate success of the social revolution depends on providing basic needs first. "If we wish for a Social Revolution, it is no doubt, first of all, to give bread to everyone…"]

B. Luxury and the fall of the anarchist Commune. [Incorrect.]

C. Freedom and the fall of the Communist system. [Incorrect. The author does not discuss freedom.]

D. Work and the hope of luxury. [Correct. The author believes the desire for luxury is ubiquitous once basic needs are met. "Still he cherishes the hope of some day satisfying his tastes more or less, and for this reason he reproaches the idealist Communist societies."]

20. According to the passage, which of the following is most likely true about the relationship between inner need and society?

A. An uncivilized society does not have to meet as many needs as an advanced society. [Correct. "…the more society is civilized, the more will individuality be developed, and the more will desires be varied." Therefore, a less civilized society will have fewer needs, according to the author.]

C. Each citizen is guided by the same fundamental desires. [Incorrect. "…the more society is civilized, the more will individuality be developed, and the more will desires be varied."]

B. The more civilized a society, the more time its citizens will have to enjoy more luxuries. [Incorrect. Time is never discussed.]

D. The members of an anarchy will have the greatest variety of needs. [Incorrect. How civilized a society is, not its form of government, decides its level of needs.]

21. According to one historical authority on the idealist Communist society, "…you suppress the possibility of obtaining anything besides the bread and meat which the commune can offer to all, and the drab linen in which all your lady citizens will be dressed." The authority would probably:

A. Agree with the author's beliefs about the social revolution. [The authority and the author agree on the criticism of Communism. But we are not given any insight about the authority's views on social revolution.]

B. Support the main critics of the author. [Incorrect. There is common ground between the authority and the author.]

C. Caution the founders of idealist societies. [Correct. This is the best answer choice. Since the authority and the author agree on the criticism of Communism, we can infer that the authority would agree with the author's criticism of founders of new societies. "These are the objections which all communist systems have to consider, and which the founders of new societies, established in American deserts, never understood."]

D. Object to the author's claim about anarchist Communes. [Incorrect.]

Answers and Explanations

22. Which of the following circumstances would the author accept as a probable explanation for the one in a hundred animals that die from old age?

A. The animal possessed greater natural strength and stamina. [Incorrect. All animals grow old and weak.]
B. The animal was near the top of the food chain. [Incorrect. The author never compares position in the food chain with surviving into old age.]
C. The animals was able to overcome all threats and attacks. [Incorrect.]
D. **The creature was lucky enough to have never faced a fatal accident. [Correct. "In that state the fullest vigor, with brightness of all the faculties, is so important that probably in ninety-nine cases in a hundred any falling-off in strength, or decay of any sense, results in some fatal accident."]**

23. Implicit in the passage is the assumption that:

A. Dying is a peaceful process. [Incorrect. This is made explicit in the passage.]
B. **Animals are without much thought. [Correct. The author believes animals experience a simple death, and never mentions agony due to thoughts. "In whatever way the animal perishes… his death is a comparatively easy one." When humans have time to think about dying, agony ensues. "The physical pain is simply nothing: the whole bitterness is in the thought that he must die."]**
C. Humans accept death when it arrives. [Incorrect. This is made explicit through example in the passage.]
D. Fear and death are separate entities. [Incorrect. This is made explicit in the passage.]

24. An editor who is critical of the author would most likely support which of the following statements?

A. **Pain is the final sensation before death. [Correct. This opposes what th author believes - neither animals nor humans necessarily feel pain right before dying. "Even when there was no loss of consciousness… they seemed not to feel it, and were, at the time, indifferent to the fate that had overtaken them."]**
B. Death from old age is very rare. [Incorrect. The author would agree with this opinion. "…will agree that death from decay, or old age, is very rare…"]
C. Physical pain from dying in cold is not significant. [Incorrect. The author would agree with this opinion.]
D. Disease is rare in wild animals. [Incorrect. The author would agree with this opinion. "As to disease, it is so rare in wild animals…"]

25. The author treats the ideas of death in animals and that in humans as distinct from each other. Which of the following characteristics supports this distinction?

A. **Pain. [Correct. Animals experience physical pain, while humans suffer from mental anguish.]**
B. Fear. [Incorrect. Both experience fear.]
C. Decay. [Incorrect. Both have the capacity to experience old age.]
D. Survival. [Incorrect. Survival was not discussed as such in the passage.]

26. According to the passage, which of the following circumstances describe a *difficult death*?

A. Two tigers attacking each other. [Incorrect. There is an enemy to fight or escape from.]
B. A soldier wounded by an enemy's blade. [Incorrect. There is an enemy to fight or escape from.]
C. A seal bleeding from a polar bear attack. [Incorrect. There is an enemy to fight or escape from.]
D. **A deer pierced by a hunter's arrow. [Correct. Here, there is no enemy to fight or escape from. "In whatever way the animal perishes, whether by violence, or excessive cold, or decay, his death is a comparatively easy one. So long as he is fighting with or struggling to escape from an enemy, wounds are not felt as wounds, and scarcely hurt him…"]**

27. What role does the idea of a cloud play in the passage?

A. It offers a symbol of calm that characterizes the nature of painless death. [Incorrect.]
B. **It reminds the reader that the source of fear is not lasting. [Correct. The cloud is used in the passage as a metaphor for the entity <u>causing</u> fear, not for fear itself. The shadow of the cloud represents fear.]**
C. It is a metaphor for fear. [Incorrect. The shadow of the cloud represents fear, while the cloud represents the temporary things that cause such fear.]
D. It offers a representation of death. [Incorrect.]

28. The passage would most likely appear in which of the following formats?

A. A report in an anthropology journal. [Incorrect. The author is not studying the origins of animals or people.]
B. **An editorial in a zoology publication. [Correct. The author most likely studies animals, and is making a comparison to humans.]**
C. A philosophical treatise on dying. [Incorrect. The emphasis is not on the philosophy of dying, but on the experience of dying comparing that of animals to humans.]
D. A sociology journal. [Incorrect. Sociology just focuses on humans, and not on animals.]

29. If excessive pressure were to build up in an old boiler that was fitted with a meter, safety valve, and no check valve, then which of the following would most likely occur?

A. An explosion. [Incorrect. This would happen without a check valve and safety valve in place.]
B. **The meter would break. [Correct. The first paragraph tells us that the check valve prevents the hot water from being forced back into the meter in case of extreme pressures.]**
C. The boiler would overheat. [Incorrect.]
D. A leak. [Incorrect.]

30. According to the passage, hot water flowing through lead pipes would most likely cause:

A. Rust formation. [Incorrect. This happens in steel pipes.]
B. **Steam formation. [Correct. "If the heat becomes more intense and steam is formed, the expansion is much greater, and some means must be provided to allow for it."]**
C. Condensation. [Incorrect. This happens in ice-water pipes.]
D. Noise. [Incorrect. This happens in clogged pipes.]

31. The author's main motivation for writing this passage is to:

A. persuade readers to use appropriate valves and materials. [Incorrect. Today's meters do not need valves.]
B. ensure that proper safety measures are in place. [Incorrect. Safety is one of several issues in the passage.]
C. **provide efficient methods of plumbing. [Correct. The author writes about ways to prevent heat loss, freezing, condensation, etc.]**
D. discuss various materials used for pipes, coverings, and storage tanks. [Incorrect. Materials are discussed, but the bigger picture is efficiency.]

32. The intended audience for this passage is most likely:

A. **Inspectors. [Correct. People who need advanced knowledge of plumbing methods to ensure safety and efficiency of piping systems.]**
B. Engineers. [Incorrect. The author does not discuss aspects of constructing pipes or materials.]
C. Manufacturers. [Incorrect. The author does not discuss aspects of constructing pipes or materials.]
D. Residents. [Incorrect. The passage discusses pipe materials, storage tanks, etc, which a home resident would most likely not change on his or her own.]

33. One can infer that cold-water pipes need covering in order to:

A. prevent crack formation. [Incorrect. The author shows concern for temperature effects first, which may then lead to cracking.]

B. reduce the rise in temperatures. [Incorrect. You want to cover cold water pipes to encourage a rise in temperature to prevent freezing.]

C. silence the noise caused by them. [Incorrect.]

D. prevent them from freezing. [Correct. Freezing would occur first, before cracking. This is the best answer.]

34. Suppose that a non-dissolvable polymer is applied to the inner lining of pipes, and that the polymer is later found to peel and dislodge. This would most likely cause:

A. Vibrations. [Incorrect.]

B. Cracking. [Incorrect.]

C. Snapping. [Correct. The non-dissolvable polymer would accumulate and clog the pipes. "When the pipes are stopped up, steam is formed and a snapping and cracking sound is heard."]

D. Faster flow. [Incorrect. Accumulation of polymer would slow down the flow.]

35. According to the passage, the following bookbinding processes most likely cause decay EXCEPT:

A. Embossing. [Incorrect. This damages books.]
B. Tanning. [Correct. Not all tanning processes are harmful. "The class of tanning materials which produce the most suitable leather for this particular purpose belong to the pyrogallol group…"]
C. Brightening. [Incorrect. This damages books.]
D. Dyeing. [Incorrect. This damages books.]

36. Bookbinders should select leather based on:
    I.   appearance.
    II.   mechanical testing.
    III.   durability testing.

A. I only [Incorrect.]
B. III only [Correct. The author does not trust absolutely the appearance nor the mechanical testing of books. The author is mainly concerned with durability.]
C. I and II only [Incorrect.]
D. I and III only [Incorrect.]

37. Which of the following, if true, would most *weaken* the author's claim that librarians are not qualified to select leather?

A. The processing of leather has become more complex. [Incorrect. This would strengthen the claim.]
B. Bookbinding is a relatively simple process. [Incorrect.]
C. Librarians are involved in the bookbinding process. [A tempting answer. The author believes librarians are not suited because of the complexity of the manufacturing process. This answer does not address this issue as well as answer D.]
D. Leather manufacturers include details of the production process in each book. [Correct. The author believes librarians are not suited because of the complexity of the manufacturing process. So if this process were clearly explained, then librarians would be qualified.]

38. The passage suggests that a librarian should consider returning a book to its manufacturer if:

A. upon mechanical testing, straight fibers are formed. [Incorrect.]
B. it is embossed using light pressure. [Incorrect.]
C. it is made with sheep skin. [Correct. "East Indian or 'Persian' tanned sheep and goat skins, which are suitable for many purposes, and are now used largely for cheap bookbinding purposes, are considered extremely bad."]
D. pages fall out. [Incorrect. No mention of pages falling out was made.]

39. The author feels confident about the durability of a book if it:

A. tears with difficulty, revealing silky fibers. [Incorrect. This tearing test does not guarantee solid durability.]
B. contains sumach. [Incorrect.]
C. **bears a hall-mark. [Correct. "Companies interested in leather, may be induced to establish a standard, and to test such leathers as are submitted to them, hall-marking those that come up to the standard."]**
D. is acid-free. [Incorrect. Acid-free paper was never discussed.]

40. Suppose that the author used a steel knife that fractured after two years of use. The author would most likely react with:

A. surprise, because steel has high tensile strength. [Incorrect. The author would not be surprised.]
B. surprise, because a knife should last longer than two years. [Incorrect. The author would not be surprised.]
C. **understanding, because repeated use ruins materials. [Correct. The author understands that just because an object may be strong, it may not resist the wearing down from use. "…it has been shown that the leather that is mechanically the strongest, is not necessarily the most durable and the best able to resist the adverse influences to which books are subject in libraries."]**
D. understanding, because durability depends on strength. [Incorrect. The author suspects that durability and strength are two separate entities..]

Verbal Test 3

Answers and Explanations

1. Suppose a new university applied for its own domain name. Problems would arise if:

A. the university allocated too many machines to act as name servers. [No. Only if too few machines were allocated would there be a problem. "The only requirements are that the requestor have two machines reachable from the Internet, which will act as name servers for that domain."]

B. the university asked another university to host its name servers. [No. Another university can host the name server as long as maintenance is dependable. "(U of I could ask Michigan State to act on its behalf and that would be fine). The biggest problem is that someone must do maintenance on the database."]

C. the root servers at the university were turned off. [Correct. The machines acting as root name servers must be on in order for outside computers to communicate with them. "The only requirements are that the requestor have two machines reachable from the Internet, which will act as name servers for that domain."]

D. too many subdomains were allocated to the domain. [No. The passage never discusses problems of over-allocation of subdomains.]

2. What is the correct relationship between names and addresses?

A. If a machine moves to a different network, the addresses will change and the name will change. [Incorrect.]

B. If a machine moves to a different network, the addresses will change but the name could remain the same. [Correct. "First, note that an address specifies a particular connection on a specific network…" Addresses point to specific connections in a network. The question requires you to make the deduction that each machine has a specific connection in a network. Thus if the location of a machine moves, then the address will change. "A name is a purely symbolic representation of a list of addresses on the network…"]

C. If the machine moves, the address moves with it. [Incorrect.]

D. Addresses are static. [Incorrect.]

3. According to the passage, if host files at the NIC did not automatically update their modification dates, then:

A. Machines would check the NIC nightly, but never download updated files. [Correct. If modification dates do not change, then the machines have no reason to download them. "Machines connected to the Internet across the nation would connect to the NIC in the middle of the night, check modification dates on the hosts file, and if modified move it to their local machine."]

B. Changes to the host file would have to be made nightly. [This is not indicated in the passage.]

C. The NIC would be overwhelmed with machines logging in constantly. [This is not indicated in the passage.]

D. Machines would not check the NIC nightly. [No. The machines would still check the NIC nightly.]

4. According to the passage, what is one possible consequence of a mistaken installation parameter?

A. Root servers will point to the wrong resolver. [This is incorrect and not supported by information in the passage.]
B. The base of the tree structured data retrieval system will be lost. [This is incorrect and not supported by information in the passage.]
C. The resolver will no longer know how to contact across the network. [No. The passage never indicates this.]
D. **A list of addresses of servers for the subdomains will not be provided. [Correct. The incorrect installation parameter will fail to indicate which root servers to use. Without the correct root servers, the resolver cannot contact the 'edu' name server which supplies it with a list of addresses of servers for the subdomains. "From the root server the resolver finds out who provides 'edu' service. It contacts the 'edu' name server which supplies it with a list of addresses of servers for the subdomains…"]**

5. The author would disagree with which of the following statements about network communication?

A. Root servers provide a list of addresses of servers for the subdomains. [Incorrect. The author indicates this to be true. "Root servers are the base of the tree structured data retrieval system… It contacts the 'edu' name server which supplies it with a list of addresses of servers for the subdomains…"]
B. The same machine can act as a server for both domains and subdomains. [Incorrect. The author indicates this to be true. "The only requirements are that the requestor have two machines reachable from the Internet, which will act as name servers for that domain. Those servers could also act as servers for subdomains…"]
C. A computer can choose which address to use for communication, as provided by the resolver. [Incorrect. The author indicates this to be true. "The user's machine then has its choice of which of these addresses to use for communication."]
D. **An allocated domain usually receives one subdomain. [Correct. The author would disagree. Once a domain is allocated, the administrator can freely allocate subdomains. "The other thing to note is that once the domain is allocated to an administrative entity, that entity can freely allocate subdomains using what ever manner it sees fit."]**

6. Suppose that the author were to teach a course, what is the most likely title for the class?

A. Root Servers 101 [Incorrect. This is too specific.]
B. How to Manage Servers [Incorrect. This is close, but the focus is not only on servers.]
C. Computers, Resolvers, and Modernization [Incorrect. This is too global. Modernization is not part of the author's discussion.]
D. **Domains and Subdomains on Campus [Correct. The passage focuses on how computers recognize servers with a focus on campus addresses.]**

7. According to the passage, which of the following is most likely to occur when the three conditions for original law are absent?

A. Only laws of nature will exist. [Incorrect. The absence of the three conditions would negate the existence of law.]

B. Law in its proper sense will have no existence. [The absence of the three conditions would negate the existence of law. "In this its strict sense the law can only exist in connection with beings possessed of reason to understand it, of power to obey it, and of free will to determine whether they will obey it or not…"]

C. Law will remain unchanged. [Incorrect.]

D. Laws of nature will remain unchanged. [Incorrect.]

8. What is the best distinction between natural law and Mr. Darwin's concept of law?

A. Darwin's concept of law pertains to civic events. Natural law pertains to observed events. [Incorrect. Civic events were never discussed.]

B. Darwin's concept of law pertains to understandable events. Natural law describes uniform events. [Incorrect.]

C. Darwin's concept of law pertains to unchangeable events. Natural law describes Divine events. [Incorrect.]

D. Darwin's concept of law pertains to the sequence of events. Natural law describes Divine events. ["Mr. Darwin… from time to time reminds us that by Nature he means nothing but the aggregate of sequences of events, or laws… It is this Will then which has its expression in the so-called laws of nature."]

9. How would the author account for Divine interference in a world that followed an original plan?

A. Designs of the Author of Nature were part of the plan from the beginning, but that the time for them had not yet come. [Yes. "But this does not preclude the possibility of Divine interference in the processes either of Creation or of Providence. New forces may from time to time be supplied, new directions may be given to existing forces, without any variation in the laws by which the action of those forces is regulated."]

B. Designs of the Author of Nature were part of a progressive act, but that the original plan had not changed. [Incorrect.]

C. Uniformity of the work might lead us to forget the Being who was working, and thus perceive the plan as unchanged. [The author does not indicate this.]

D. Nature follows an aggregate of sequences of events, which is recognized as Divine interference. [Incorrect.]

10. The author would most likely agree with which of the following statements about conscious acts?

A. Conscious acts involve deciding which forces to call forth and in what manner, influencing laws of nature. [Not supported.]
B. Conscious acts ascend from our own works to those of God. [The author never indicated this.]
C. Conscious acts operate in a certain prescribed manner that directs human will. [This is not the best answer.]
D. Conscious acts operate on predictable natural forces that cannot interrupt natural laws. [Correct. "But in all these cases there is no interruption of the law by which the working of these forces is regulated. We have then a limited control over these forces, and yet they are unchangeable in themselves, and in their mode of action."]

11. Suppose that an astronomer discovers that Nature operated like a predictable machine. If true, how would this statement change the meaning of Nature according to the author?

A. The true meaning of the word would be lost. [Correct. The author makes the argument that Nature is not simply a sequence of events.]
B. The meaning of the word would not change. [Incorrect. The meaning would change because it goes against the meaning proposed by the author.]
C. The meaning of Nature would expand to include natural events. [No.]
D. The meaning of Nature would be complete. [Never indicated.]

12. The passage suggests that according to the original sense of the word, Nature was the expression of:

A. natural sequences of events. [Not the best answer.]
B. natural phenomenon made by a Creator of order and uniform procedure. [The author believes Nature describes natural phenomenon, and a Creator of order created it.]
C. natural forces operating in a prescribed manner. [Not the best answer.]
D. natural phenomenon open to influence. [Not the best answer.]

13. Which of the following statements, if true, would most *weaken* the study of the manors of the Bishopric of Winchester?

A. Tenants refused to take up land on old terms at the onset of the Black Death, but did so prior to the pestilence. [Correct. The Bishopric of Winchester study found that key changes, such as tenants not wanting to take up land on old terms, began long before the onset of the Black Death.]
B. Villains were obtaining concessions from their lords prior to the Black Death. [Incorrect. This supports the study.]
C. Landowners did not face serious difficulties during the Black Death, but did so prior to the pestilence. [Incorrect. The study acknowledges temporary changes took place during the pestilence, so this answer would not weaken the study.]
D. The temporary increase in economic burden caused by the Black Death was one reason for the ability of the villains of the decade 1350-1360 to enforce their demands. [Incorrect. Not relevant.]

14. The passage supports each of the following statements about the Black Death EXCEPT:

A. Serfs desired to improve their social status. [Incorrect. "The serfs who had survived the pestilence took advantage of the opportunity afforded by their reduction in numbers to free themselves from servile labor and thus improve their social status."]
B. Changes in manorial management were gradual. [Incorrect. "The connection between the Black Death and the changes in manorial management which are usually attributed to it could be more convincingly established had not several decades elapsed after the Black Death before these changes became marked."]
C. Landowners used less force to secure holders for bond land after the pestilence. [Correct. "Before the Black Death landowners were unable to secure holders for bond land without the use of force. A generation after the Black Death they were still contending with this problem, and it had become more serious than at any previous time…"]
D. Changes in the tenure of land occurred prior to the pestilence. [Incorrect. "The Black Death at the most did no more than accelerate changes in the tenure of land which were already under way."]

15. The author would most likely *disagree* with which of the following statements:

A. The pestilence does not explain the events which took place long after its effects were forgotten. [The main argument of the passage is that the changes seen during the Black Death were well underway before the pestilence, and continued long after the pestilence.]
B. The Black Death can explain a condition which arose before its occurrence. [Correct. The author is arguing against this]
C. One result of the pestilence was to place villains in a stronger position than before. [Yes. The author argues this point using the Levett and Ballard explanation.]
D. Landowners were already facing serious difficulties before 1348. [Yes. The author argues this point using the Levett and Ballard explanation.]

16. Which of the following does the author consider to be a temporary effect during the mid-fourteenth century?

A. The reduction in the number of serfs. [Yes. "The strength of the position of the serfs lay not so much in the absence of competition due to a temporary reduction in their numbers as in their poverty."]
B. The concessions obtained by villains. [Concessions existed well before the Black Death. "…but without the help of any such cause, villains of an earlier period were obtaining concessions from their lords,"]
C. The worthlessness of the land. [This was chronic. "The absence of competition for holdings was no temporary thing, due to the high mortality of the years 1348-1350, but was chronic, and was based upon the worthlessness of the land."]
D. The absence of competition for holdings. [This was chronic. "The absence of competition for holdings was no temporary thing, due to the high mortality of the years 1348-1350, but was chronic, and was based upon the worthlessness of the land."]

17. Villains were able to secure lower rents by using:

A. poverty as an excuse to refuse services. [Yes. "Villains were refusing to perform their services on account of poverty, and they were already securing reductions in their rents and services."]
B. force against landowners. [Incorrect. Landowners used force.]
C. economic burdens as leverage against serfs. [Never stated.]
D. the worthlessness of land as a means to shorten their tenure of the land. [Never stated.]

18. One would best characterize the field of occupation of the author as being:

A. political. [Incorrect. While the author may be an attorney, there is a clear element of education present.]
B. legal. [Incorrect. While the author may be an attorney, there is a clear element of education present.]
C. educational. [Correct. The overall purpose is to educate the reader about some possible misconception about the Black Death.]
D. agrarian. [Incorrect. While the author may be an attorney, there is a clear element of education present.]

19. What is the main idea of the Canopus and Rigel example?

A. We cannot conclude that because a star is bright, it is near. [Yes. "Perhaps the attribute in which the stars show the greatest variety is that of absolute luminosity. The most striking example of this is afforded by the absence of measurable parallaxes in the two bright stars, Canopus and Rigel, showing that these stars, though of the first magnitude, are immeasurably distant…"]

B. Parallax cannot measure with reliability the distance of a star. [Incorrect. The Canopus and Rigel example demonstrated that we cannot correlate brightness with nearness.]

C. Spectroscopic examination can apply to both near and distant stars. [No.]

D. The distances of Canopus and Rigel are immeasurably great. [True, but not the main point of the example.]

20. The author most likely views the analogy between stellar statistics and sociology as

A. appropriate, because both fields classify members by accounting for them individually. [Not the best answer.]

B. imperfect, because stellar statistics cannot account for every planet. [Correct. The author explains this. "In the field of stellar statistics millions of stars are classified as if each taken individually were of no more weight in the scale than a single inhabitant of China in the scale of the sociologist. And yet the most insignificant of these suns may, for aught we know, have planets revolving around it, the interests of whose inhabitants cover as wide a range as ours do upon our own globe."]

C. apropos, because both fields deal with immense numbers. [May be true, but ignores the difference between the two.]

D. unbalanced, because stellar statistics does not include all the interest of the human race. [No. The author does not expect stellar statistics to include all the interest of the human race.]

21. The synthesis of spectroscopic examination, luminosity, and stellar statistics would be most similar to the study of

A. glowing beetles in a state park. [No. The number of beetles in a park can be counted. The better analogy is one that presents a vast number of objects.]

B. refraction of light through raindrops. [No. Refraction is not made of particles or objects.]

C. luminescent algae in the ocean. [Yes. The correct answer must demonstrate an innumerable amount of the object, and a signal given off by the object that can vary in strength (preferably light). The object must be countable.]

D. solar wind encountering the Earth's atmosphere. [No. Solar wind cannot be counted.]

22. According to the passage, the Milky Way is composed primarily of stars with:

A. a shade of yellow, scattered through a spherical space of unknown dimensions, but concentric. [Incorrect.]
B. greater absolute brilliancy, and rather slower in motion. [Yes. "These are distinguished from the others by being bluer in color, generally greater in absolute brilliancy, and affected, there is some reason to believe, with rather slower proper motions."]
C. a shade of blue, composing the great girdle, and faster in motion then stars in the spherical region. [Incorrect.]
D. slower motion and less brilliance than stars in the spherical region. [Incorrect.]

23. The author would LEAST agree with which of the following observations:

A. The patterns of stellar luminosities support the outcome of Kapteyn's conclusions. [This is not supported by the passage.]
B. Relatively speaking, the sun can be considered a dim or bright star. [Yes. Nearness does not mean a star will be bright or dim necessarily.]
C. Observations reveal no motion in Rigel. [True. "Rigel has no motion that has certainly been shown by..."]
D. Apparent motions depend on distance. [This is supported in the passage. "...apparent motions, as ordinarily observed, these are necessarily dependent upon the distance of the star."]

24. The author suggests that spectroscopic examination:

A. Could detect different velocities of stars in the girdle and sphere of the Milky Way. [Incorrect.]
B. Would be applicable to the field of sociology. [This is never suggested.]
C. Could show two stars at different distances as having the same velocities. [Yes. "Spectroscopic examinations seem to show that all the stars are in motion, and that we cannot say that those in one part of the universe move more rapidly than those in another."]
D. Could reveal the distances of stars. [No. "But the results of spectroscopic measurements of radial velocity are independent of the distance of the star."]

25. According to the passage, the Democrats and Republicans would most likely agree on each of the following EXCEPT:

A. taxes on corporations. [Irrelevant. Never discussed in the passage.]
B. immigration. [Both agree. "Republicans attempted to throw a sop to the labor vote by favoring restriction of immigration and laws... The Democrats went even further..."]
C. **valuable land ownership. [Correct. Democrats went further than Republicans on the land ownership issue. "The Democrats went even further and demanded the return of 'nearly one hundred million acres of valuable land' then held by 'corporations and syndicates, alien and domestic.'"]**
D. the standard money of the country. [Both agree. "Said the Democratic platform: 'We hold to the use of both gold and silver as the standard money of the country, and to the coinage of both gold and silver without discrimination against either metal or charge for mintage.' The rival Republican platform declared that 'the American people, from tradition and interest, favor bimetallism...'"]

26. As implied by the passage, Harrison was most likely running on which ticket?

A. Populist. [No.]
B. **Republican. [Yes. "In Minnesota the Populists, with a ticket headed by the veteran Donnelly, ran a poor third in the state election, and the entire Harrison electoral ticket was victorious in spite of the endorsement of four Populist candidates by the Democrats."]**
C. Democrat. [No.]
D. Independent. [Never stated.]

27. What is the main idea of the passage?

A. The 1890s saw the emergence of a new U.S. political party. [No. Too general.]
B. The Populist party evolved under the leadership of Weaver. [Too narrow an answer.]
C. The Democrats and Republicans influenced the emergence of the new Populist party. [This is true, but the emphasis should be on the Populist Party, not the other parties.]
D. **The Populist party emerged with questionable success. [Yes. The passage is about the Populist party and its struggles to succeed.]**

28. According to the passage, the Populist Party was most successful in which region of the United States?

A. Iowa and Missouri. [Not as strong as other regions.]
B. Illinois. [A Democrat won here.]
C. California. [No. "On the Pacific coast, despite the musical campaign of Clark, Mrs. Lease, and Weaver, California proved deaf to the People's cause;"]
D. Minnesota. [Correct. "In the northwestern part of the State, however, the new party was strong enough to elect a Congressman over candidates of both the old parties."]

29. The passage is most likely:

A. a transcript from a documentary. [Yes. The formal tone and educational nature of the passage fits well with a transcript from a documentary.]
B. an editorial from a local newspaper. [No. An editorial contains opinionated language.]
C. an article in a business journal. [No. The focus is not business.]
D. a report from the Populist Party. [No. The article takes a third-person point of view with respect to the political parties.]

30. According to the passage, the inventor of a significant theorem must possess which of the following qualifications?

A. quick perception of detail [Not the best answer.]
B. complete knowledge of mathematical science [Incorrect. Knowledge of the mathematical science is not enough.]
C. flair for creativity [Correct. "At the time of the discovery of the beautiful theorem of Huygens, it required in its author not merely a complete knowledge of the mathematical science of his age, but a genius to enlarge its boundaries by new creations of his own."]
D. interest in mankind [Not the best answer.]

31. In the context of the passage, the word *ornaments* most nearly means:

A. scientists [Too specific. Ornaments may refer to more than just scientists.]
B. laity [Too specific. Ornaments may refer to more than just laity.]
C. priests [Too specific. Ornaments may refer to more than just priests.]
D. members [Correct. Ornaments may refer to scientists, laity, and priests.]

32. In organizing a society to maximize the number of ideas put to practical use, the author would most likely advise:

A. the government to offer tax relief to all inventors in the society. [More reward should be given to the founders of ideas.]
B. academic institutions to offer professorships to only the inventors of ides. [False. More reward should be given to the founders of ideas.]
C. that a percentage of profits be given to the inventors of ideas on which product are based. [Correct. "Unless there exist peculiar institutions for the support of such inquirers, or unless the Government directly interfere, the contriver of a thaumatrope may derive profit from his ingenuity, whilst he who unravels the laws of light and vision, on which multitudes of phenomena depend, shall descend unrewarded to the tomb."]
D. that profits be given to the inventors of useful applications that came from abstract ideas. [No. More reward should be given to the founders of ideas.]

33. Which of the following statements, if true, would support the author's point about rewarding the originators of ideas?

A. Government profits as much from the invention as does the public. [No. A lack of reward to those who come up with the theories and ideas upon which inventions are made is the problem.]
B. Government is able to judge fully the merit of the invention. [Incorrect for the same reason.]
C. Rewards from the sale of the invention are not given to the inventor. [Yes. A lack of reward to those who come up with original theories and ideas upon which inventions are made is the problem.]
D. Government bestows a greater reward than that which arises from the sale of the commodity to the public. [Incorrect for the same reason.]

34. Which of the following statements would the author find most surprising?

A. Universities have a history of creating new ideas. [Correct. "Perhaps it may be urged, that sufficient encouragement is already afforded to abstract science in our different universities, by the professorships established at them. It is not however in the power of such institutions to create"]
B. The inventor of the crossbow had complete knowledge of mechanical physics, and the genius of creating a more portable device. [Not the best answer choice.]
C. Hundreds of years passed between the invention of the wheel, and that of the chariot. [A large amount of time would not necessarily surprise the author.]
D. Most inventors of ideas are not supported by their governments. [The author would not find this surprising.]

35. A *thaumatrope* most likely refers to:

A. a box that emits a specific pitch of sound when light shines on it. [No. This does not use light and vision.]
B. a mechanical violin played by turning a crank. [No. This does not use light and vision.]
C. a glass bulb of mercury that rises or falls based on humidity. [No. This does not use light and vision.]
D. a card with a picture on each side that is twirled quickly. [Correct. This is the only invention that utilizes light and vision. "…or unless the Government directly interfere, the contriver of a thaumatrope may derive profit from his ingenuity, whilst he who unravels the laws of light and vision, on which multitudes of phenomena depend, shall descend unrewarded to the tomb."]

Answers and Explanations

36. The author's central thesis is that:

A. The business of farming fosters individualism. [No. This is too broad.]
B. Farmers develop a state of mind unfavorable for organization. [No. This strays from the main idea.]
C. **The Grange is the most successful effort to unite the farming class. [Correct. The passage is about the Grange.]**
D. The Grange was born of two needs. [No. Too specific.]

37. According to the passage, the Grange derives much of its credibility from:

A. the early rush to the Grange. [Incorrect. "The truth of this statement will immediately be questioned by those whose memory recalls the early rush to the Grange…"]
B. its broad membership. [No. This was not discussed.]
C. publications. [No. "The truth of this statement will immediately be questioned … by those whose impressions have been gleaned from reading the periodicals…"]
D. **its near national status. [Correct. "Not only is it at the present time active, but it has more real influence than it has ever had before; and it is more nearly a national farmers' organization than any other in existence today."]**

38. According to the passage, the assertion "The Grange is dead" was not true because:

A. **it achieved more than any other farm organization. [Yes. "The Grange has accomplished more for agriculture than has any other farm organization."]**
B. it is still active. [No. While this is true, it is not the main refutation of the quote.]
C. it is the oldest general organization for farmers. [No. While this is true, it is not the main refutation of the quote.]
D. it reversed the tide of isolation in the farming community. [No. This was not mentioned.]

39. The passage implies each of the following statements about rural organization EXCEPT that:

A. it faced much struggle in its origins. [This is true. "…and that the weapons of rural organization have a temper all the better, perhaps, because they were fashioned on the anvil of defeat."]
B. brotherhood now exists between North and South. [This is implied. "…and the immediate need was that of cultivating the spirit of brotherhood between the North and the South. The latter need no longer exists; but the fundamental need still remains and is sufficient excuse for the Grange's existence today."]
C. **great progress has been made. [Correct. This is not implied, because it is stated directly. "But it is also true that great progress has been made…"]**
D. organizations previous to the Grange never reached full national status. [This is implied. "Not only is it at the present time active, but it has more real influence than it has ever had before; and it is more nearly a national farmers' organization than any other in existence today."]

40. The example of O. H. Kelly best illustrates the point that:

A. nobody would help agriculturalists except for its own members. [Correct. Kelly realized that politicians would never help the farmers. "On this tour he became impressed with the fact that politicians would never restore peace to the country; that if it came at all, it would have to come through fraternity."]

B. farmers called for a secret society of agriculturists. [Incorrect. The idea began with Kelly, not the community.]

C. fostering kindly feelings among farmers was the first step towards a solid union. [No. This is not stated.]

D. the agricultural masses became suspicious of one another. [This is stated in the passage, but the example of Kelly is not relevant.]

VERBAL TEST 4

ANSWERS AND EXPLANATIONS

1. In order to identify a person to be a great leader of society, the author would most likely look for the
    following qualities EXCEPT:

    **A. congeniality. [Correct. The author gives examples of rulers who do not possess congeniality, so we
    do not expect the author to look for this trait in a ruler. "…some great rulers have been
    unintelligible like Cromwell, or brusque like Napoleon, or coarse and barbarous like Sir Robert
    Walpole."]**
    B. audacity. [The author would expect this trait in a ruler based on the examples given. "By boldness, by
    cultivation, by "social science" they raise themselves above others."]
    C. temperance. [The author would expect this trait in a ruler based on the examples given. "George III had
    no social vices, but he had no social pleasures. He was a family man, and a man of business, and sincerely
    preferred a leg of mutton and turnips after a good day's work to the best fashion and the most exciting
    talk."]
    D. cultivation. [The author expects this trait in leaders. "By boldness, by cultivation, by "social science" they
    raise themselves above others."]

2. Suppose the author decided that a head of society were a natural idea for a particular country. Whom
    would the author advise to lead this country?

    A. The head of civil government. [Incorrect.]
    B. The chair of religious affairs. [This is never indicated in the passage.]
    C. The president of a business. [Not the best answer.]
    **D. The director of a social club. [The author points out that society is the union of people for
    amusement and conversation. "Society, in the sense we are now talking of, is the union of people for
    amusement and conversation."]**

3. Which of the following claims is (are) explicitly presented in the passage to justify the supposition that
    society does not naturally need a head?
    I.   The top level of society naturally overtakes a political leader.
    II.   Organization for communication differs from organization for religious purposes.
    III.   Despite the presence of a Monarchy, society resorts to oligarchic organization.

    A. I only [The passage does not support this.]
    **B. III only [Correct. "In consequence, society in London, though still in form under the domination of
    a Court, assumed in fact its natural and oligarchical structure. It, too, has become an "upper ten
    thousand"; it is no more monarchical in fact than the society of New York."]**
    C. I and II only [The passage does not offer these as justification for the supposition that society does not
    naturally need a head.]
    D. I, II and III [No.]

4. The author of the passage would support most probably an England where:

A. a King would be the figurehead, and the highest citizens would run the country as political officials. [The author sees no natural reason to have a head at all.]

B. a King would run the entire country. [The opposite is supported by the passage.]

C. no King would exist, and the highest citizens would run the country as political officials.[Correct. "In the first place, society as society does not naturally need a head at all. Its constitution, if left to itself, is not monarchical, but aristocratical... . There is nothing in this which needs a single supreme head; it is a pursuit in which a single person does not of necessity dominate."]

D. all citizens would have equal voting power. [No. The author believes in an aristocracy.]

5. Which of the following statements, if true, would most *weaken* the author's approval of the French Government?

A. The Emperor promotes himself to higher levels of status and power. [The author suggests that the people of France elevate their own king. This answer is incorrect for the additional reason that it would not weaken the author's approval of the French Government.]

B. The Court of France maintains veto power over the Emperor. [No.]

C. A lower class does, in fact, exist in France at this time. [This is irrelevant to the question.]

D. Class distinctions broaden as the head of France gains power. [Correct. The author approves of the theory of equality in France. "The theory of his Government is that every one in France is equal, and that the Emperor embodies the principle of equality. The greater you make him, the less, and therefore the more equal, you make all others."]

6. Suppose that a citizen of France were asked to compare the Emperor to the Queen of England. The citizen would most likely mention that:

A. The Emperor has the divine right to promote himself more so than does the Queen. [Incorrect. This was not clearly spelled out.]

B. The Queen may lead the state, but the Emperor is the state. [Correct. This is straight from the passage. "The Emperor represents a different idea from the Queen. He is not the head of the State; he IS the State."]

C. The Queen is not as powerful as the Emperor. [Incorrect. This is implied and not the best answer.]

D. The Emperor is like God, while the Queen is mortal. [Incorrect. This was never mentioned.]

7. The author would find which of the following most objectionable?

A. A child whining and pretending to cry to persuade others. [Correct. The author disapproves of anyone feigning emotion to win over others.]
B. A policeman yelling at an attacker to cease and desist. [No.]
C. An animal growling for no apparent reason. [Incorrect. The author would not find this objectionable.]
D. A fog horn signaling ships on a clear day. [Incorrect.]

8. How would the author complete the following thought? "One of the great mistakes of our religious life is our…"

A. blind trust in clergy. [A tempting choice, but it does not capture the full meaning of the author's objection.]
B. pursuit of progressive culture. [Incorrect.]
C. mistaking noise for religion. [Correct. The author complains that congregations are getting caught up with the noise of church, and not its message. "It is true, perhaps, that in most of our congregations large numbers of people love to hear the "tone," but when and how are the people ever to become acquainted with higher religious ideas?"]
D. desire to get ahead. [This is mentioned, but is not the main concern.]

9. The author places the blame for "retarding the religious progress of the race" on the:

A. ministers. [No. The author places blame on the congregation as well.]
B. church attendees. [No. The author places blame on the ministers as well.]
C. selfish pursuits. [Incorrect.]
D. ministers and church attendees. [Yes. Both are to blame. "Our educated ministers are making a serious mistake… It is true, perhaps, that in most of our congregations large numbers of people love to hear the 'tone'…"]

10. In the passage "the welkin ring" most nearly means:

A. a circle of believers holding hands. [Incorrect.]
B. a wedding ring. [Incorrect.]
C. a very loud sound. [The author makes reference to the welkin ring where sound is a concern. You are not expected to know the true meaning of the welkin ring, and must infer it. "they become infatuated with certain tones and give vent to their "feelings" by making the welkin ring."]
D. a bobbin for weaving. [Incorrect.]

11. The author's argument in the final paragraph compared to the criticism expressed in the earlier portion of the passage is:

A. **ironic. [Correct. In the final paragraph, the author denounces the nature of people to pull each other down. "If one attempts to gain a certain goal, there always stands another ready to pull him back." The fact that the author is criticizing ministers with such force earlier in the passage is ironic.]**
B. satirical. [The author is not satirical.]
C. sarcastic. [The author is not sarcastic.]
D. critical. [The author is critical, but his dual criticisms create a tone of irony.]

12. Each of the following statements about ministers is NOT supported by the passage EXCEPT:

A. They are aware of their potentially displeasing styles, and believe some people do not desire them. [Incorrect.]
B. **They are aware of their potentially displeasing styles, but believe some people desire them. [Correct. The ministers admit to their high-flown ways, and acknowledge that some members desire it. "The mourning preachers will admit in private that there is no virtue in the mourn, and that they do it simply to 'touch up' the old folks."]**
C. They are unaware of their potentially displeasing styles, but believe some people desire them. [Incorrect.]
D. They are unaware of their potentially displeasing styles, and believe some people do not desire them. [Incorrect.]

13. The author would most likely compare the experience of the "unthinking classes" attending church to:

A. **watching a soap opera. [Correct. The author talks about the appeal to emotion as the key compelling force for the unthinking class. A soap opera appeals to emotion. "Instead of carrying home some practical thought and trying to weave it into their lives, they become infatuated with certain tones and give vent to their "feelings" by making the welkin ring."]**
B. attending a circus. [Incorrect.]
C. playing a sport. [Incorrect. The appeal is not to a competitive spirit.]
D. going to sleep. [Incorrect.]

14. The author would explain the long neck of a giraffe most likely by:

A. using the theory of evolution as a model. [Incorrect. The author tells us that evolution alone cannot explain many adaptations.]

B. studying the complete genealogy of giraffes. [No. The author turns to the causes and conditions, not the genealogy.]

C. explaining why the animal needs it. [No. The author tells us that simply explaining adaptations based on needs is not sufficient. "If we are asked why the elephant has a trunk, we must answer because the animal needs it. But does such a reply in itself explain the fact? Evidently not."]

D. examining the causes and conditions that led to the long neck. [Correct. "We must determine the causes and conditions that have cooperated to produce this particular result if our answer is to constitute a true scientific explanation."]

15. The main idea of the mechanistic position is that:

A. adaptations often seem to contradict mechanical conditions. [No. This would contradict the mechanistic position.]

B. nature is crammed with devices to protect and maintain the organism. [May be true, but is not the best answer.]

C. adaptations are mechanical responses to the environment. [Correct. The mechanistic position believes adaptations are direct results of environmental pressures.]

D. the body has functional adaptations. [This is true, but not the best answer choice.]

16. Each of the following examples represents a structural adaptation that a "mechanist" can readily interpret, EXCEPT:

A. A flatworm cut into two pieces, and each grows into two identical new flatworms. [No. The mechanist is challenged with adaptations that must change in response to a changing environment.]

B. A lizard losing its tail, and growing a new one. [No. The mechanist is challenged with adaptations that must change in response to a changing environment.]

C. A frog using different lungs to breathe in water or on land. [No. The mechanist is challenged with adaptations that must change in response to a changing environment.]

D. An octopus that changes color for camouflage. [Correct. "He has a far more difficult knot to disentangle in the case of the so-called functional adaptations, where the organism modifies its activities (and often also its structure) in response to changed conditions."]

17. The attitude of the author towards the concept of "vital force" is best described as:

A. neutral. [Incorrect. The author has an opinion on the matter.]
B. skeptical. [Incorrect. The author does not doubt or attack the existence of the vital force, but simply questions its validity.]
C. **speculative. ["Shall we find anything corresponding to the usual popular conception— which was also along the view of physiologists—that the body is "animated" by a specific "vital principle," or "vital force," … that exists only in the realm of organic nature? If such a principle exists, then the mechanistic hypothesis fails and the fundamental problem of biology becomes a problem sui generis."]**
D. curious. [No.]

18. Based on information in the passage, the author would support each of the following statements EXCEPT:

A. The living body is a machine. ["It is not open to doubt that the living body is a machine."]
B. **Adaptations follow mechanical conditions. [Correct. The author wishes to point out that the mechanistic view of adaptations is incomplete.]**
C. Science must look beyond why things exist. ["The question which science must seek to answer, is how came the elephant to have a trunk…"]
D. Physiologists believe the body is animated. ["Shall we find anything corresponding to the usual popular conception—which was also along the view of physiologists—that the body is "animated"…]

19. Suppose the lens of an animal's eye, after it is removed, regenerates perfectly but from a different layer of cells than those of the original lens. How would the author respond to this finding?

A. Acknowledge it as support of the mechanistic viewpoint. [Incorrect.]
B. **Be astounded by it, and offer no valid explanation. [Correct. The author views adaptations as arising from environmental pressures. In the case of the lens regenerating from a new set of cells, there is no pressure from the environment causing this to happen. Thus, we would expect the author to be astounded.]**
C. Suspect it to be erroneous. [Incorrect. The passage never indicates this.]
D. Accept it as support of evolution. [Incorrect. In fact, such a finding may cause the author to favor the vital force theory.]

20. The discussion of the Protestant Revolution shows primarily that:

A. celibacy ceased to be a sign of righteousness. [This is too specific.]
B. several radical ideas emerged as a consequence. [This is too vague.]
C. women had to break with the traditions that defined their position. [Most of the passage is not about how women broke from traditional roles.]
D. it went far to restore respect for women. [Correct.]

21. According to one historian, the French Revolution taught freedom from authority among men and women. If true, the French people would view marriage most likely as a(an):

A. outmoded ceremony. [This is never suggested in the passage.]
B. simple union between man and woman. [Correct. The passage states that beliefs cannot be destroyed by revolution, but the question stem indicates the French Revolution taught freedom from authority among men and women. So the correct answer is one that incorporates both ideas – marriage is not forgotten, but is not maintained as a sacred ceremony. "But beliefs cannot be directly destroyed by revolution; they can only be disturbed and modified…"]
C. sacrament. [No. The passage never indicates that people do not listen to the messages of a revolution.]
D. legal bond. [Incorrect. Legality is never discussed.]

22. According to the passage, how were women treated in the American colonies?

A. With full freedom and opportunity. [No. The passage states that women did not enjoy full freedom. "Why then did not the American Revolution pass on to full freedom and opportunity for women?"]
B. Conservatively, with new opportunities. [Correct. "In fact, the student of colonial records finds many traces of ultra conservatism in the treatment of women, though the forces had been liberated which must inevitably open the way for her through the New World of America into a new world of the spirit."]
C. With few freedoms. [No. The passage suggests that women had many freedoms, but not full freedom. "Why then did not the American Revolution pass on to full freedom and opportunity for women?"]
D. In a very restricted fashion, yet with a fresh spirit. [Not the best answer.]

23. The author suggests that each of the following factors motivated women to seek freedom EXCEPT:

A. intemperance. ["Miss Susan B. Anthony also began her public life as a teacher and a temperance reformer."]

B. intolerance from men. ["It was only when she found herself helpless, in presence of the prejudices against her sex, that she turned her attention to freeing women from all purely sex limitation in public life."]

C. dissatisfaction with the status of marriage. [Correct. This is never suggested in the passage.]

D. injustices existing after the Civil War. ["In the Civil War, women directly served men; but in the great industrial reorganization which came afterward they served mainly women and children. Here the victories have been won in the press, in the legislative halls, and in courts of law. Working with men, or alone, they have perfected organization, agitated, raised money, printed appeals, and carried cases through the courts…"]

24. According to the passage, women did not have full access to opportunities following the American Revolution. How would the author most likely explain this?

A. Many improvements occurred, but the image of women as subordinate to men dominated society during this time. [Incorrect. This is an attractive answer choice, but the passage makes no reference to the image of women.]

B. Women did not fight hard enough for effective change, and lost the freedoms they enjoyed during Colonial America. [The passage tells us that women did fight hard for change, and enjoyed an expanded role after the Civil War.]

C. Despite the many interest and momentous changes, only the most imperative needs could receive attention. [Interests were so numerous that only the most pressing needs received the attention of the people. "Why then did not the American Revolution pass on to full freedom and opportunity for women? For the same reason that it did not forever abolish slavery in America. The vested interests involved were so many, and the changes so momentous and difficult…"]

D. The abolition of slavery overshadowed the Women's Movement. [An attractive answer, but nothing in the passage suggests this.]

25. The passage suggests that the most favorable portrayal Sir George Campbell gave of Falling in Love was to interpret it as:

A. the best interest of the race. [Sir George Campbell does not think highly about Falling in Love.]
B. a universal selective process. [Not the best answer.]
C. skin deep. [This is a better choice than A or B, but his ideas about Falling in Love go beyond skin deep.]
D. **psychological folly. [Correct. "Sir George Campbell's conclusion is exactly the opposite one from the conclusion now being forced upon men of science by a study of the biological and psychological elements in this very complex problem of heredity. So far from considering love as a foolish idea."]**

26. Suppose Sir George Campbell announced that beauty is one of the very best guides we can possibly have to the desirability of any man or any woman as a partner in marriage. How would this information affect the author's claims about modern biology?

A. It would support the claim that modern biology causes people to seek their moral, mental, and physical complement. [The concept of beauty as a selection factor is emphasized in the biological selection process in paragraph 4.]
B. It would weaken the claim that modern biology causes people to fall in love in particular places and particular societies they happen to be cast among. [No, it would not weaken the claim.]
C. **It would support the claim that modern biology follows a ubiquitous selection process. [Correct. The author defends Falling in Love as a process that follows a biological selection process that emphasizes beauty, strength, and health. "Falling in Love, as modern biology teaches us to believe, is nothing more than the latest, highest, and most involved exemplification, in the human race, of that almost universal selective process... We do fall in love, taking us in the lump, with the young, the beautiful, the strong, and the healthy."]**
D. It would weaken the claim that modern biology protects love as an essentially beneficent and conservative instinct developed and maintained in us by natural causes. [No, it would not weaken the claim.]

27. The passage suggests that, before the time of physiologists and psychologists of the modern evolutionary school, experts regarded the act of Falling in Love as:

A. a conservative instinct. [No. This is what competent physiologists and psychologists of the modern evolutionary school think.]
B. **foolish and not useful. [Correct. The author suggests that physiologists at some time in the past considered love as a foolish idea. "So far from considering love as a 'foolish idea,' opposed to the best interests of the race, I believe most competent physiologists and psychologists, especially those of the modern evolutionary school, would regard it rather as an essentially beneficent and conservative instinct"]**
C. not clearly beneficial. [This is a tempting choice, but ignores the suggestion that physiologists at some time in the past considered love to be a foolish idea.]
D. a controllable, deliberate process of selection. [Incorrect.]

28. The passage as a whole suggests that in order to find true love, people must:

A. fall in love with their counterpart. [Not the best answer.]
B. seek out their true complement. [Not the best answer.]
C. meet someone of opposite constitution who appeals to their innermost nature. [Correct. The passage explains that the most valued partner will appeal to one's inmost nature. "But among the women he actually meets, a vast number are purely indifferent to him; only one or two, here and there, strike him in the light of possible wives, and only one in the last resort (outside Salt Lake City) approves herself to his inmost nature as the actual wife of his final selection."]
D. fall in love with someone of the same class in society. [Falling in love with someone of the same class does not guarantee the person will appeal to their innermost nature.]

29. The tone of the author towards Sir George Campbell can be best described as being:

A. satirical and instructive. [Correct. The author is exposing Sir George Campbell to some mild ridicule while being informative and persuasive.]
B. smug, yet polite. [The author is not smug.]
C. disapproving and ironic. [The author disagrees with Sir George Campbell, but does not necessarily disapprove of him. Irony is also not present.]
D. blithe, yet critical. [The author is not showing a lack of concern. This is irrelevant.]

30. According to the passage, men and women fall in love:

A. in the class they find themselves in. [Correct. "Men and women as a rule very sensibly fall in love with one another in the particular places and the particular societies they happen to be cast among."]
B. with someone who pays much attention to the other person. [Incorrect. This is probably true, but not the strongest answer.]
C. when biology determines it to happen. [Incorrect. This is not the best answer.]
D. unexpectedly. [Incorrect.]

31. Which of the following statements weaken the argument of the author?

    I.   If the balance of energy of a tidal wave were to become disrupted, the tides would cease.

    II.   If tidal energy were utilized by engineers, the machines driven would be driven at the expense of the earth's rotation.

    III.   Hot air currents in Earth's atmosphere cause the rotation of Earth to slow ever so slightly.

A. I only [No. The author would probably agree with this statement.]

B. III only [Tides, not air, are causing the slowing down. "The energy of the tides is, in fact, continually being dissipated by friction, and all the energy so dissipated is taken from the rotation of the earth."]

C. I and III only [Incorrect.]

D. I, II and III [Statement II is not a correct answer because it does not address a key point of the author that tides are causing the Earth's rotation to slow.]

32. Suppose that in 7,200 years, a solar eclipse will occur on Earth. Compared to today, a place on the Earth's surface will come into the shadow:

A. 4 hours late. [Incorrect]

B. 2 hours early. [Incorrect. The Earth is slowing down, not speeding up.]

C. 2 hours late. [Correct. The passage tells us that the earth's rotation is slowing down 1 hour every 3,600 years. Compared to today, 7,200 years into the future will mean that a point on the Earth's surface will appear 2 hours behind where it should be.]

D. 3 hours early. [Incorrect]

33. A supporter of the theory about Mars and its moon would most likely believe that the Earth will:

A. collide eventually with the moon. [Yes. "Mars is therefore slowly but surely pulling its moon down on to itself..."]

B. draw closer but never collide with the moon due to the pull of neighboring planets. [No.]

C. be pulled further apart from the moon. [Opposite to what is stated.]

D. increase its rate of spin, and retard the revolution of the moon. [Never indicated.]

34. This passage would most likely appear in what format?

A. newspaper [The passage is too scientific to appear in a newspaper.]

B. letter from the editor in a journal [The passage does not have a conversational style.]

C. academic lecture [Yes. The sophistication and erudite language is appropriate here.]

D. textbook [The passage contains philosophical language that does not fit best in a textbook.]

35. Each of the following statements is supported by an explanation or example in the passage EXCEPT:

A. Mankind is capable of recognizing eternity. ["No less are we compelled to recognize the existence of incalculable eons of time, and yet to perceive that these are but as drops in the ocean of eternity."]
B. The length of day of Mars' moon is increasing. ["…but its tides are following its moon more quickly than it rotates after them; they are therefore tending to increase its rate of spin, and to retard the revolution of the moon."]
C. A distant, yet massive planet will have the same effect on tides as a smaller, closer planet. [Correct. This is not mentioned in the passage.]
D. If a solar eclipse thirty-six centuries ago was an hour early, then a place on the earth's surface came into the shadow one hour ahead of time. [Yes, because this is the reverse of what is stated. "The statement that a solar eclipse thirty-six centuries ago was an hour late, means that a place on the earth's surface came into the shadow one hour behind time."]

36. Which statement, if true, would most *weaken* the argument of the secessionists?

A. **Sovereignty vests not in the States severally, but in the States united, or that the Union is sovereign, and not the States individually. [Correct. The secessionist argument rests on the supposition that sovereignty rests on "the original and inherent rights of the several States as independent sovereign States…" If sovereignty no longer applies to independent States, but only to States united, then the argument comes apart.]**
B. The Union is not a firm, a copartnership, nor an artificial or conventional union. [This would strengthen the secessionist argument, not weaken it.]
C. Sovereignty vests in the States severally, and the Union is a partnership. [This does not weaken the argument as strongly as answer A does.]
D. The Union, like a firm, has the power to compel its members to remain. [This would weaken the argument of the secessionists, but makes no reference to the sovereignty of individual States.]

37. The author uses the example of Roman jurisdiction to make which point about territories in the United States?

A. A territory of the United States is automatically a part of the nation's political population. [Not supported by the passage.]
B. **A territory can be subject to the United States, but makes no part of the political population until admitted into the Union. [Correct. This parallels the example of Roman jurisdiction in the passage. "The provincials were subjects of Rome, but formed no part of the Roman people, and had no share in the political power of the state, until at a late period the privileges of Roman citizens were extended to them, and the Roman people became coextensive with the Roman Empire…"]**
C. A territory cannot be subject to the United States without redefining its boundaries. [Not the best answer.]
D. A territory of the United States becomes admitted into the Union when privileges of US citizens are extended to it. [A tempting answer, but choice B is more accurate.]

38. The author would view the citizens of states who revolt for secession as:

A. revolutionists. [Tempting, but this word may have a negative connotation which the author would not normally attribute to these citizens.]
B. sovereign citizens. [True, but this answer misses the full meaning of how the author would view these citizens.]
C. traitors. [No. This is the opposite of the correct answer.]
D. **patriots. [Correct. Since the people are citizens, the author would defend their right to revolt for secession. "There is no power in a firm to compel a copartner to remain a member any longer than he pleases… the original and inherent rights of the several States as independent sovereign States."]**

39. Referring to the thirteen states of the original United States as mentioned in the final paragraph, suppose nine states ratify the constitution and four do not. How would the author view the status of the states that refuse to sign?

A. The four states step beyond their rights and competency. [Incorrect.]
B. The four become independent sovereign States. [No. The States would default to territories.]
C. **The four states default to territories under the Union. [Correct. The author believes territories have no sovereign power apart from the Union. So, by refusing to enter the Union these States would remain territories under the Union. "The Territory gives up no sovereign powers by coming into the Union, for before it came into the Union it had no sovereignty, no political rights at all. All the rights and powers it holds are held by the simple fact that it has become a State in the Union."]**
D. The four states become privately held territories. [Cities can become private owners of territory, but the passage gives no information about private ownership of states.]

40. The author would most likely support all of the following statements EXCEPT:

A. The Union does not have jurisdiction over the whole population who live in the United States. [The author would agree. "But this one sovereign people that exists only as organized into States, does not necessarily include the whole population or territory included within the jurisdiction of the United States."]
B. **The State relinquishes its rights when it enters the Union. [Correct. The author does not acknowledge the rights of territories, but does so for States. Thus, the author would not support a claim that States relinquish their rights. "All the rights and powers it holds are held by the simple fact that it has become a State in the Union."]**
C. The Union is not formed by the surrender to it by the several States of their respective individual sovereignty. [The author does not believe that States surrender their sovereignty when joining the Union.]
D. Provincials are subjects of a nation and do not necessarily comprise its people. [The author would agree. "But this one sovereign people that exists only as organized into States, does not necessarily include the whole population or territory included within the jurisdiction of the United States."]

VERBAL TEST 5

ANSWERS AND EXPLANATIONS

1. Which statement about Plato's concept of government is incorrect?

A. The polity is less perfect than Plato's previous constructs. [This concurs with Plato's concept of government. "…his whole plan of government neither a democracy nor an oligarchy, but something between both, which he calls a polity… but if he intended it to be the next in perfection to that which he had already framed, it is not so…"]

B. Governance should not include tyranny. [Plato's Laws does offer one form of government that is composed of a democracy and a tyranny. So choice B is correct. "It is also said in this treatise of Laws, that the best form of government must, be one composed of a democracy and a tyranny.."]

C. Monarchies are not of serious consideration. [This concurs with Plato's concept of government. "But now in this government of Plato's there are no traces of a monarchy, only of an oligarchy and democracy…"

D. Governance tends towards oligarchies. [This concurs with Plato's concept of government. "But now in this government of Plato's there are no traces of a monarchy, only of an oligarchy and democracy; though he seems to choose that it should rather incline to an oligarchy, as is evident from the appointment of the magistrates…"]

2. The political state described in the final paragraph:

A. mimics the Lacedaemonian form of government. [This is not supported by the passage.]

B. reduces the power of the senate. [There is no evidence for this. This is not supported by the passage.]

C. will not consist of a mix between a democracy and a monarchy. [Correct. The final paragraph depicts a political state where many of the commonality will not vote in elections, and the state will be run by the first rank of senators. Thus, the state will not be a democracy nor a monarchy.]

D. gives the majority of control to the magistrates. [No. It will give the majority of control to senators.]

3. All of the following forms of government were described in the passage EXCEPT:

A. a combination of democracy, oligarchy, and monarchy. [This is in the passage. "Some persons say, that the most perfect government should be composed of all others blended together, for which reason they commend that of Lacedaemonian; for they say, that this is composed of an oligarchy, a monarchy, and a democracy…"]

B. a combination of democracy and oligarchy, without any monarchy. [This is in the passage. "But now in this government of Plato's there are no traces of a monarchy, only of an oligarchy and democracy…"]

C. a combination of democracy and monarchy, without any oligarchy. [Correct. The author makes no mention of this combination.]

D. a semi-democracy and semi-oligarchy. [This is the polity. "Now he is desirous to have his whole plan of government neither a democracy nor an oligarchy, but something between both, which he calls a polity."]

4. According to the author, what do ephori and polity have in common?

A. some essence or form of democracy. [Correct. Both contain elements of democracy. "Now he is desirous to have his whole plan of government neither a democracy nor an oligarchy, but something between both, which he calls a polity… that in the ephori may be found the democratical, as these are taken from the people."]

B. guardianship by men-at-arms. [Men-at-arms are found in the polity, and not in the ephori.]

C. approval from the senate. [The author never talks about senatorial approval of either the ephori or polity.]

D. absolute power. [Absolute power applies only to ephori.]

5. Which of the following circumstances favors democracy over oligarchy?

A. When all commoners are obliged to vote for senators of all four classes. [Correct. In this case all people will vote, and there will be an equal number of senators of each rank.]

B. A king is elected by popular vote by all people. [An attractive answer, but not discussed in the passage.]

C. Commoners vote for their own representatives in a Lacedaemonian form of government. [This is not explained in the passage.]

D. Senators from the third and fourth classes vote for representatives from the commonality. [An attractive answer, but not discussed in the passage.]

6. According to the passage, how will the average genius writer approach the task of writing about sailing for two separate newspapers?

A. The writer will write with a style that catches the tone of one newspaper, and then change the style of the article to catch the tone of the other newspaper. [Correct. The author indicates that most men of genius will write according to what is expected of them, which includes conforming to the style of a given publication. "…most men of genius are susceptible and versatile, and fall into the style of their age…What writers are expected to write, they write; or else they do not write at all…"]

B. The writer will write with a style that departs from the tone of one newspaper, and then change the style of the article to catch the tone of the other newspaper. [Incorrect. The average genius writer will not use a style that departs from a target publication.]

C. The writer will write two different articles using the same tone in each piece, and submit them to the newspapers. [Incorrect.]

D. The writer will submit the same article to both newspapers. The style of the article will differ from the style of either newspaper in order to create a new style. [Very few genius writers can forge a new style.]

7. The passage implies that a new writer emerges from competing writers when:

A. The new writer mimics the style of a currently famous author. [No. Imitating a style does not create a new style.]

B. The new writer unconsciously imitates the style of a currently famous author. [No. Imitating a style does not create a new style.]

C. The new writer is bold enough to break through and create a style of his own. [A tempting choice, but does not go far enough. Simply writing a new style does not guarantee wide receptivity and the emergence of a new writer.]

D. The new writer's style imprints itself upon the memories of people more so than that of other writers. [Correct. In order for men to like the words before them, they must remember what they enjoy. When one style makes a lasting impression, then that style will become more popular. "Many men—most men—get to like or think they like that which is ever before them, and which those around them like, and which received opinion says they ought to like; or if their minds are too marked and oddly made to get into the mold, they give up reading altogether, or read old books and foreign books, formed under another code and appealing to a different taste."]

8. According to the passage, under what circumstances would an original Nonconformist writer become an original Conformist writer?

A. When the Nonconformist writer, sensing a shift in the popular style, changes his style to meet that shift. [No. This would cause the Nonconformist to become an unoriginal Conformist.]
B. When the popular style happens to shift to a style that matches that of the Nonconformist. [Correct. In this case the writer maintains his originality while becoming a seemingly Conformist writer.]
C. When the popular style happens to shift away from the Conformist's style. [No. This is incorrect.]
D. When the Conformist writer, sensing a shift in the popular style, fails to change his style to meet that shift. [This would not cause an original Nonconformist writer to become an original Conformist writer.]

9. The tone of the author is best described as:

A. instructive. [Incorrect. The author is not instructing the reader.]
B. insensitive. [Incorrect.]
C. sympathetic. [Incorrect.]
D. persuasive. [Correct. The author is trying to persuade us to agree on the various kinds of writers.]

10. Suppose it was discovered that national character emerges in a similar fashion to that of popular literary style. How would the author describe the emergence of America's national character?

A. A chance predominance of character arising from colonial life, and the society unconsciously imitating it. [Correct. This parallels the emergence of popular literary style. A certain style happens to arise, and most writers imitate it.]
B. A predominance of character arising from a political leader in colonial life, and the society unconsciously imitating it. [No.]
C. A chance predominance of character arising from colonial life, and the political leader of the society imitating it. [No. The society must unconsciously imitate it.]
D. A predominance of character arising from a political leader in colonial life, and the future elected leaders imitating it. [Incorrect. The society must imitate it.]

11. How would the author best describe human instinct?

A. The human mind tends to mimic what is around it. [Not the best choice.]
B. The human spirit has an innate tendency to break from popular style. [This opposes what the author feels about most writers.]
C. The human mind has an inherent desire to mimic a mold, whether that mold is imposed or not. [Yes. As exemplified by writers, people tend to imitate a mold that may or may not be imposed.]
D. The human spirit will not peruse something that is not popular. [The passage suggests that the human spirit will peruse what is popular. The contrapositive is not necessarily true.]

Answers and Explanations

12. Suppose that professors were making public proclamations that computers would never be able to beat a human being in chess. How would hackers respond to this claim?

A. They would reject the claim and attempt to build the best chess program possible. [Correct. Hackers had no boundaries. "Hackers felt otherwise: anything that seemed interesting or fun was fodder for computing—and using interactive computers, with no one looking over your shoulder and demanding clearance for your specific project, you could act on that belief."]

B. They would consider a chess program a misappropriation of valuable machine time. [Incorrect. This is the standard thinking at the time, not representative of hackers.]

C. They would remain quiet to maintain their positions in academia. [Incorrect. The passage never talks about hackers remaining quiet.]

D. They would build a bug to beat a human player. [Incorrect. A bug is an accidental fault in a program. Hackers would not purposely build a bug.]

13. Which of the following, if true, would most likely change the author's attitude towards the Hacker Ethic?

A. Programs built by hackers benefit computers. [This would not change the author's attitude. The author knows that hackers build programs that somehow further mankind.]

B. Hackers write programs in FORTRAN. [This would be of no consequence to the author, and is thus the wrong answer choice.]

C. Hackers create programs that harm users of computers. [Correct. The author approves of the Hacker Ethic because it benefits the world. So if hackers made programs that did harm to people, the author would no longer support it. "And wouldn't everyone benefit even more by approaching the world with the same inquisitive intensity, skepticism toward bureaucracy, openness to creativity, unselfishness in sharing accomplishments, urge to make improvements, and desire to build as those who followed the Hacker Ethic?"]

D. Hackers create bugs inadvertently which have unpredictable consequences. [The author already knows this, and does not have a big concern about it.]

14. Suppose a hacker built a program for a Mars rover to drive around obstacles on the ground. How would the program work?

A. The rover would stop in front of the obstacle, evaluate the best path, reject other paths, and use parameters to choose the ultimate path. [No.]

B. The rover would stop in front of the obstacle, evaluate paths around it, reject the longest path, and use parameters to choose the ultimate path. [No.]

C. The rover would stop in front of the obstacle, evaluate the best path, reject the longest path, and use parameters to choose the ultimate path. [Incorrect.]

D. The rover would stop in front of the obstacle, evaluate paths around it, reject most, and use parameters to choose the ultimate path. [Correct. This most closely parallels the passage. "It took a while (everyone knew that during those pauses the computer was actually 'thinking,' if your idea of thinking included mechanically considering various moves, evaluating them, rejecting most, and using a predefined set of parameters to ultimately make a choice)."]

15. The following statements are supported by the author EXCEPT:

A. Kotok spent years building the chess program. [This is supported. "Kotok kept at it for years, the program growing as MIT kept upgrading its IBM computers…"]

B. Without floating-point arithmetic, the program will not know where to place the decimal point. [This is supported. "After two or three months of tangling with intricacies of floating-point arithmetic (necessary to allow the program to know where to place the decimal point)…"]

C. A bug caused one pawn to jump over another pawn. [This is supported. "Finally, the computer moved a pawn two squares forward—illegally jumping over another piece."]

D. Wagner used assembly to build a computer program. [Correct. The author does not specify which program Wagner used.]

16. The author is most likely a:

A. hacker. [Correct. The author's strong support of the Hacker Ethic suggests that the author is a hacker.]

B. chess player. [No. There is not support for this.]

C. mathematician. [Not the best answer. The author suggests otherwise: "According to the standard thinking on computers, their time was too precious that one should only attempt things which took maximum advantage of the computer, things that otherwise would take roomfuls of mathematicians days of mindless calculating."]

D. computer scientist. [This may be true, but the passage never discusses computer scientists. The best answer is choice A.]

17. The passage as a whole suggests that in order for a plant to grow without soil, it must:

A. possess spines and thick leaves, grow on rocks, and be exposed to rain from time to time. [Some plants, as evidenced by the salicornia example, can live in sand. Growing on rocks is not the necessary alternative to soil.]

B. grow on rocks, possess a prickly covering, and survive without a drop of water. [Growing on rocks is not the only alternative to soil.]

C. grow new plants after being scattered, survive long periods without a drop of water, and possess needles. [Correct. "…desert plants… have often to struggle on through long periods of time without a drop of water... and each one terminating in a sharp, needle-like spine, which effectually protects the weed against all browsing aggressors… a marked characteristic of the cactus tribe to be very tenacious of life, and when hacked to pieces, to spring afresh in full vigor from every scrap…"]

D. multiply rapidly, retain moisture, and be exposed to rain from time to time. [To grow without soil, like desert plants, the organism must survive long periods of drought.]

18. The claim that higher organisms pay a penalty for their extreme complexity is based mainly on the:

A. examinations of sea life and desert life. [Correct. This refers to the first paragraph. The author uses the examples of the hydra, lobster, and lizard.]

B. studies of lizards and lobsters. [This excludes the hydra.]

C. observations of desert plants and animals. [This is too vague and excludes the sea life examples.]

D. analyses of lobsters, lizards, and prickly pears. [Incorrect.]

19. The salicornia is cited in the passage as support for the inference that:

A. many shore weeds of the intermediate sand-belt mimic to a surprising degree the chief external features of the cactuses. [Correct. "That belt of dry beach that stretches between high-water mark and the zone of vegetable mold, is to all intents and purpose a miniature desert. True, it is watered by rain from time to time; but the drops sink in so fast that in half an hour, as we know, the entire strip is as dry as Sahara again… One such weed, the common salicornia, which grows in sandy bottoms or hollows of the beach, has a jointed stem, branched and succulent… and entirely without leaves or their equivalents in any way"]

B. many shore weeds have a tendency to produce rounded stems and leaves. [The salicornia is cited to draw a comparison to cactuses which do not have rounded stems and leaves.]

C. many shore weeds below the zone of vegetable mold are similar to the prickly pear. [This answer does not define the zone adequately because it excludes the lower boundary, namely the high-water mark.]

D. many shore weeds above the high-water mark have in them the ability to rebuild in its entirety another organism. [This answer does not define the zone adequately because it excludes the upper boundary, namely the zone of vegetable mold.]

20. Which of the following statements, if true, would most *weaken* the conclusions of the author?

A. True vegetable hydras, when you cut down one, ten spring in its place. [The author would agree with this.]
B. Every separate morsel of thick and succulent stems of desert plants has the power of growing into a separate cactus. [This would not weaken the main thrust of the passage.]
C. The prickly pear is designed for its fruit to be devoured by birds and animals. [This is not relevant.]
D. All plants in regions starved of rain survive by accessing underground water. [Correct. This fact would weaken the close correlation between water-preserving adaptations and arid environments, suggesting the superfluous nature of such adaptations.]

21. As suggested by the passage, which of the following features are characteristic of most plants and animals?

      I.   Defense mechanisms to not get eaten.
      II.   The tendency to preserve water.
      III.   The power to regenerate in its entirety another organism.

A. I only. [Yes, but III is also correct.]
B. II only. [The tendency to preserve water is discussed in relation to plants, but not to animals.]
C. I and III only. [Correct. "Yet, even among animals, at a low stage of development, this original power of reproducing the whole from a single part remains inherent in the organism… and to set at defiance the persistent attacks of all external enemies… As far as their leaf-like stems go, the main object in life of the cactuses is—not to get eaten."]
D. II and III only. [Statement II is not correct.]

22. The tone of the author is best described as:

A. ironic. [No.]
B. curious. [No.]
C. instructive. [The author is not only instructive in tone, but also interested.]
D. fascinated. [Correct. The author takes interest in the subject.]

23. In the context of the passage, the word *best* means:

A. hybridize. [Incorrect.]
B. defeat. [Correct. Man has managed to overcome the survival mechanisms of the plant. "The more you cut it down, the thicker it springs… Man, however, with his usual ingenuity, has managed to best the plant, on this its own ground, and turn it into a useful fodder for his beasts of burden."]
C. isolate. [No.]
D. remove. [A tempting answer, but this section of the passage focuses on plant survival. Thus, 'defeat' is a better answer.]

Answers and Explanations

24. The author indicates that many forms of government exist because:

A. each form arose from essentially an oligarchy or democracy. [Not supported by the passage.]

B. there are many forms of magistracies, since they control governments. [This does not answer the question. Just because an answer choice is true, it may not answer the question.]

C. each state is made up of many kinds of citizens, which governments are meant to serve. [A tempting choice, but D captures the idea that states comprise many different parts.]

D. each state consists of a great number of parts. [Correct. The passage states this clearly. "It is evident then, that there must be many forms of government, differing from each other in their particular constitution: for the parts of which they are composed each differ from the other."]

25. If the power of a state were to be distributed according to the beauty of its citizens, the state would be:

A. a republic. [No.]

B. an aristocracy. [The author focused on democracy and oligarchy near the end of the passage.]

C. a democracy. [Since beautiful people comprise the minority of a population, the state would be an oligarchy.]

D. an oligarchy. [Correct. Beautiful people comprise the minority of a population, so the state would be an oligarchy. "We should rather say, that a democracy is when the supreme power is in the hands of the freemen; an oligarchy, when it is in the hands of the rich: it happens indeed that in the one case the many will possess it, in the other the few; because there are many poor and few rich."]

26. Which of the following statements, if true, would most *weaken* the author's concept of governance?

A. A democracy is a state where the poor are invested with ruling power, and an oligarchy is a state where noble families are invested with ruling power. [This would not weaken the argument.]

B. A democracy is a state where the poor are invested with ruling power, and an oligarchy is a state where the freemen are invested with ruling power. [This would not weaken the argument.]

C. A democracy is a state where noble families are invested with ruling power, and an oligarchy is a state where the poor are invested with ruling power. [This is the correct answer because it opposes the author's concept of governance. The author views a democracy as government of the many, and an oligarchy as government of the few. "And thus in politics, there is the government of the many and the government of the few; or a democracy and an oligarchy…"]

D. A democracy is a state where noble families are invested with ruling power, and an oligarchy is a state where the beautiful are invested with ruling power. [This answer fails because the second part about oligarchy might support the views of the author.]

27. The main idea of the passage is that:

A. government is a just and fair form of social contract. [Not the best answer.]
B. out of two integral forms of government come all other forms. [A tempting choice, but choice D is better since it takes into consideration the author's emphasis on the correlation between size of ruling party and government type.]
C. as there are various kinds of people in society, there are various forms of government. [This is too general, and a trap answer.]
D. **governments are some variant of two essential forms, determined by the size of the ruling party. [Correct. The author views music as he does governments – that all forms derive from two essential forms. "…to distinguish governments as I have done, into two species: one, of those which are established upon proper principles; of which there may be one or two sorts: the other, which includes all the different excesses of these…"]**

28. The author of the passage would probably agree with each of the following statements about government EXCEPT:

A. **A democracy occurs when the supreme power is lodged in the people. [Correct. The author states explicitly that a democracy should not be defined by this condition. "We ought not to define a democracy as some do, who say simply, that it is a government where the supreme power is lodged in the people; for even in oligarchies the supreme power is in the majority."]**
B. An oligarchy is like a discordant melody. [The author would support this. "…the oligarchic and despotic to the more violent tunes…"]
C. Several forms of government derived from the oligarchic form. [The author would support this. "…distinguish governments as I have done, into two species: one, of those which are established upon proper principles; of which there may be one or two sorts: the other, which includes all the different excesses of these…"]
D. If the poor acquired power over the rich, then a democracy could possibly form. [The author would support this. "We should rather say, that a democracy is when the supreme power is in the hands of the freemen; an oligarchy, when it is in the hands of the rich: it happens indeed that in the one case the many will possess it, in the other the few; because there are many poor and few rich."]

29. Which of the following findings best supports the author's belief that rural schools should become social centers?

A. Rural schools are not as strong as they should be in history, writing, reading, the sciences and other subjects. [No. Never indicated.]

B. Students in rural schools are drifting from the life of farm community. [Yes. "History, writing, reading, the sciences, and even other subjects can be taught so as to connect them vitally and definitely with the life of the farm community."]

C. Rural schools are like machines. [No. This is a concern, but not the main motivator.]

D. The School Improvement League requires schools to become social centers. [No. The need for social centers has created the League.]

30. The author of the passage would probably veto most strongly a federal law that:

A. prohibits the rural schools from shortening the total number of school days per year. [No. The author wants schools to move away from turning out students too quickly.]

B. requires parents of students to visit the rural schools on a periodic basis.[No. The author favors closer ties between home and school.]

C. assigns to rural schools additional funding for art. [No. The author favors the School Improvement League which supports art in schoolrooms.]

D. grants teachers the right to keep the progress of students private from parents to protect students. [Yes. The author advocates closer ties between schools and parents.]

31. The existence of which of the following phenomenon would most strongly challenge the information in the passage?

A. A rural school on the social center paradigm that fosters competition. [No. This is not a direct challenge to the social center concept.]

B. A graduate of the social center paradigm who abandons farm life. [No. A student leaving farm life does not challenge the worth of the social center paradigm.]

C. Nature-study produces students who are averse to collaboration. [Yes. A main goal of nature-study is to foster cooperation among students.]

D. Parents stop sending their children to rural schools on the social center paradigm. [No. There may be other factors why this could happen. It does not necessarily implicate the effectiveness or worth of the social center paradigm.]

32. According to the passage, which of the following items is(are) values of social centers?
    I. Correct observation.
    II. Immediate improvement.
    III. Quality of buildings.

A. I only [No. All three are valued.]
B. II only [No. All three are valued.]
C. I and III only [No. All three are valued.]
D. I, II and III [Yes. "The value of nature-study is recognized not only in thus making possible an intelligent study of the country child's environment, but in teaching a love of nature, in giving habits of correct observation... This means that the pupils as a body can co-operate for certain purposes, and that this co-operation will not only secure some good results of an immediate character, results that can be seen and appreciated by everyone... The purposes of the league are: (1) to improve school grounds and buildings..."]

33. The passage suggests that the cooperation between the home and school is brought about by:

A. Parents visiting the schools often. The teacher knowing more about the home life of her pupils, and the parents knowing far more about the school. [Yes. "A third method is through co-operation between the home and the school, between the teacher and pupils on one side, and parents and taxpayers on the other side."]
B. Joint meetings of teachers and school officers. [No. This does not go far enough.]
C. The teacher knowing more about the home life of her pupils, and the students knowing far more about the school. [No. Students do not need to know more about the school.]
D. Joint meetings of students and school officers. [No. The problems is a lack of connection between parents and schools].

34. The author most probably advocates each of the following EXCEPT:

A. New studies in the nature-study paradigm over old studies. [Correct. "But it is not so much a matter of introducing new studies—the old studies can be taught in such a way as to make them seem vital and human."]
B. Teaching correct observation of nature. [Incorrect. The author favors this. "...but in teaching a love of nature, in giving habits of correct observation..."]
C. Preparing students for the study of science. [Incorrect. The author favors this. "...and in preparing for the more fruitful study of science in later years."]
D. Fostering a foundation of intellectual thinking. [Incorrect. The author favors this. "...because it will show the possibilities of living an intellectual life upon the farm."]

35. The overall theme of the passage is that:

A. imitation pearls are rather difficult to detect. [Too specific.]
B. the distinction between natural and artificial pearls is difficult to make. [May be true, but is too specific.]
C. imitation pearls have several classes and means of detection. [May be true, but ignores the concept that pearls can be produced naturally.]
D. pearls can be produced naturally or artificially. [Correct.]

36. According to the passage, how do cultured pearls and natural pearls compare?

A. The time during which the oyster forms a cultured pearl is greater than is required for the growth of a large natural pearl. [Cannot say for sure.]
B. The number of layers of pearly material is greater in the cultured pearl than the number of layers of a natural pearl. [Not necessarily.]
C. The appearance of the cultured pearl is never equal to that of a fine true pearl. [The passage does not tell us this.]
D. More scales of small North Sea fish are required to make a cultured pearl then those required to make a natural pearl. [True. Scales are not required to make a natural pearl.]

37. Suppose a pearl collector wanted to distinguish Roman pearls from contemporary Indestructible pearls. How could the collector make this clear and unmistakable distinction?

A. Heat the two pearls. [Correct. The wax on the inside of the Roman pearl will melt. The newer indestructible pearls will not melt.]
B. Look for nacre on Roman pearls. [Both contain nacre.]
C. Use a magnifying glass. [Both contain the same material on the outside.]
D. Put the pearls in a glass of water. [Differences in densities is too difficult to discern in a glass of water.]

38. How would a collector estimate the age of an imitation pearl?

A. Bisect the pearl and count the number of pearly layers. [The number of layers does not change with age.]
B. Look for signs of dirt on the pearl, inside the pearl where the string passes, or on the string itself. [Correct. "Like fine natural pearls, the fine imitations should be wiped after use and carefully put away. They should also be restrung occasionally, as should real pearls both to prevent loss by the breaking of the string and because the string becomes soiled after a time, and this hurts the appearance of the jewel."]
C. Apply a force-measuring instrument to its surface to evaluate durability. [The integrity of the surface does not correlate with age.]
D. Bisect the pearl and count the number of opalescent glass layers. [The number of layers does not change with age.]

39. The article from which this passage derives would most likely appear in:

A. a journal for gem collectors. [Correct. This is the most likely answer.]
B. a government report on the pearl trade. [A government report would use more official language.]
C. an editorial in a trade journal for jewelry. [A likely answer, but editorials often contain more opinionated language.]
D. a newspaper op-ed piece. [Incorrect.]

40. One can infer that the properties of imitation pearls differ from those of natural pearls in each of the following ways EXCEPT:

A. specific gravity. [No, because the two pearls are made of different materials.]
B. degree of hardness. [No, because the two pearls are made of different materials.]
C. degree of iridescence. [Correct. They resemble each other in iridescence. "The artificial pearl thus resembles the true pearl in the physical causes for the beautiful effect."]
D. magnified surface characteristics. [Surface characteristics other than iridescence most likely differ. Also, this answer does not specify which characteristics it refers to.]

Verbal Test 6

Answers and Explanations

1. What is the main idea of the passage?

A. Milk is not prepared well enough for human consumption. [Not the best answer. The main idea is that many methods exist to best prepare milk for consumption.]
B. More methods must be discovered to prepare milk for human consumption. [No. The main idea is that many methods exist to best prepare milk for consumption.]
C. Milk safety begins with bacterial control. [Not the best answer. Some portions of the passage do not relate to bacteria. The main idea is that many methods exist to best prepare milk for consumption.]
D. **Many methods exist to treat milk for human consumption. [Correct. The author considers several methods to treat milk.]**

2. The passage implies that one hazard of preparing milk for consumption could be:

A. **overheating, which creates poor taste. [Correct. "If milk is heated for some minutes to 160° F, it acquires a cooked taste…"]**
B. forming too many fat globules. [Incorrect. The danger is in changing the aggregation of fats. "…it becomes thinner in consistency or "body," a condition which is due to a change in the grouping of the fat globules."]
C. introducing viruses. [No. The passage never mentioned viruses.]
D. poisoning by mercury salts. [No. Mercury salts are not used in milk for human consumption, so there is no danger of poisoning by this means.]

3. According to the passage, which of the following statements about the growth of bacteria is most accurate?

A. A maximum temperature exists that prevents growth. [No. A minimum temperature exists that prevents growth.]
B. **Just because bacterial organisms stop dividing does not mean they are dead. [Correct. "A temperature above the maximum growing-point (105°-115° F.) and below the thermal death-point (130°-140° F.) will prevent further growth, and consequently fermentative action."]**
C. Bacteria in milk exist primarily in spore forms. [A tempting answer, but not entirely correct. Bacteria can exist in vegetative forms too. "This temperature varies, however, with the condition of the bacteria, and for spores is much higher than for vegetative forms."]
D. Above the maximum growing-point, bacteria does not cause milk to change. [False. The temperature must reach above the death-point to stop all changes. "A temperature above the thermal death-point destroys bacteria, and thereby stops all changes."]

4. The author would disagree with each of the following statements EXCEPT:

A. Heated milk is not adequate for making cheese. [The author would disagree with this statement. "Heating milk causes the soluble lime salts to be precipitated, and as the curdling of milk by rennet (in cheese-making) is dependent upon the presence of these salts, their absence in heated milks greatly retards the action of rennet."]

B. Violations of cleanliness or cold preservation contribute mostly to bacterial changes in milk. [This is supported in the passage, and thus the author would agree with this statement. "Whenever serious difficulties do arise, attributable to bacterial changes, it is because negligence has been permitted in one or both directions."]

C. Milk should always be kept chilled once drawn from the animal until consumption. [Incorrect. If milk happens to be contaminated, it should be heated to kill bacteria. "A temperature above the thermal death-point destroys bacteria, and thereby stops all changes."]

D. People have little say in the control of milk. [The author would disagree with this statement. "…but great improvement over existing conditions could be secured if the public would demand a better supervision of this important food article."]

5. The author would most likely agree with which of the following statements about treating milk?

A. Mild forms of poisons are no longer used in the treatment of milk. [False. "…a number of milder substances are more or less extensively employed, although the statutes of practically all states forbid their use."]

B. Treating milk with heat arose after the discovery of chemical treatment. [False. The passage implies the opposite. "Heat has long been used as a preserving agent. Milk has been scalded or cooked to keep it from time immemorial."]

C. Treating milk with chemicals affects its lime salt content. [Not enough information is given in the passage to conclude this. Thus, it cannot be true.]

D. Milk dealers who use clean and cooling methods for drawing milk rarely encounter bacterial problems. [This is the best answer. "If the milk is properly drawn from the animal in a clean manner and is immediately and thoroughly chilled, the dealer has little to fear as to his product. Whenever serious difficulties do arise, attributable to bacterial changes, it is because negligence has been permitted in one or both directions.."]

6. Which natural sense, if greatly enhanced, would be most effective in preventing the occurrence of impostors?

A. Movement. [Motion is not a method of discernment.]

B. Texture. [All beings are lines, so texture cannot apply.]

C. Smell. [Smell was never discussed.]

D. Hearing. [Correct. If hearing is greatly enhanced, then beings will be able to detect the small differences among voices. "Amongst our lowest orders, the vocal organs are developed to a degree more than correspondent with those of hearing, so that an Isosceles can easily feign the voice of a Polygon, and, with some training, that of a Circle himself."]

7. According to the passage, which of the following is most likely to be true about how various beings appear in Fog?

    I.   The Circle will always appear as a straight line with a bright center.

    II.   The Square will always appear as a straight line with a bright center.

    III.   All Polygons always appear as a straight line with a bright center.

A. I only [True. Looking at a circle from the side would show a curve with a brighter middle portion.]

B. II only [No. The Square can appear to be a vertical straight line of uniform luminosity (without a bright center).]

C. II and III only [No. The Square does not always appear with a bright center.]

D. I, II, and III [Incorrect.]

8. According to the passage, how would the Physician appear?

A. A line with a bright center, but the lines of its sides recede less rapidly in the fog and will thus appear less dim as those of the Merchant. [Correct. The angles of a pentagon are wider than those of an equilateral triangle, so the arms of the angle of a pentagon recede less rapidly away from the observer.]

B. A line with a bright center, but the lines of its sides recede more rapidly in the fog and will thus appear dimmer than those of the Merchant. [Incorrect.]

C. A line with a dimmer center, while the lines of its sides will appear as dim as those of the Merchant. [Incorrect.]

D. A line with a brighter center, while the lines of its sides will appear as dim as those of the Merchant. [Incorrect.]

9. A likely title for this written piece is:

A. Geometry in a Flat World. [Incorrect. The passage is not about geometric shapes, but beings living in a flat world.]
B. Flatland, the Life. [Correct. The emphasis is on beings living in a flat world.]
C. Journey in Spaceland. [No. Ignores the emphasis on a flat world.]
D. Hearing and Sight in a Flat World. [A tempting choice, but the passage is about identifying beings in a flat world and not about mere hearing and seeing abilities.]

10. Suppose a physician were afflicted with rheumatism and his brain was registered at 95 degrees. After five generations making a full recovery, to what degree would his brain return?

A. 60 degrees. [Incorrect. This is the normal angle for an isosceles triangle. The physician is a pentagon.]
B. 98 degrees. [Incorrect.]
C. 108 degrees. [Correct. The passage tells us that a full recovery returns the being to its normal angle, as indicated in the final paragraph. The passage also tells us that the physician is a pentagon ("...we will suppose, a Merchant and a Physician, or in other words, an Equilateral Triangle and a Pentagon, respectively..."), so we must compute the normal internal angle of a pentagon using the equation provided in the passage. The angles of a pentagon are 108 degrees ((180x5 – 360)/5 = 108). Therefore, a full recovery will bring the physician back to his usual 108 degrees.]
D. 120 degrees. [No.]

11. Each of the following statements is supported in the passage EXCEPT:

A. Silent resignation is a common mode of disapproval. ["...and whilst instances of opposition amongst them have been very rare, a silent resignation to circumstances has been the most usual mode of meeting measures they disapproved."]

B. Individuals have supported all the measures of the party. [Correct. "That each individual has invariably supported all the measures of the party, is by no means the case..."]

C. Remonstrance is not well tolerated by the Council. ["If any member of the Society, feeling annoyed at the neglect, or hurt by the injuries or insults of the Council, show signs of remonstrance, it is immediately suggested to him that he is irritated, and ought to wait until his feelings subside..."]

D. Even after an interval of time has passed will a complaint be discredited by the Council. ["...if it is then brought forward, the immediate answer is, The affair is out of date—the thing is gone by—it is too late to call in question a transaction so long past..."]

12. According to the author, a better election system would consist of:

A. private nominations by the President. [The author criticizes this approach.]

B. a symposium to review nominees. [Correct. "If these lists were, as in other scientific societies, openly discussed in the Council, and then offered by them as recommendations to the Society, little inconvenience would arise; but the fact is, that they are private nominations by the President, usually without notice, to the Council, and all the supporters of the system which I am criticizing, endeavor to uphold the right of this nomination in the President, and prevent or discourage any alteration."]

C. open discussion by the Society. [No. The author does not suggest this is a better election system.]

D. a forum of discussion led by the President. [No. The author does not suggest this is a better election system.]

13. According to the passage, after a member of the Society cools off and brings forth an offense again, the reaction to him would be:

A. Recognition, since he has waited for an interval. [Incorrect.]

B. Acceptance, since he has calmed down. [No, because acceptance does not follow.]

C. Disregard, since he was irritated. [No, because the person has calmed down.]

D. Dismissal, since the offense has expired. [Correct. "...if it is then brought forward, the immediate answer is, The affair is out of date—the thing is gone by—it is too late to call in question a transaction so long past."]

14. The existence of which of the following procedures would most strongly challenge the information in the passage?

A. The Society's consideration of an offense by a member of the Council. [This could happen according to the author.]
B. The party opposing all improvements to the Society. [Incorrect.]
C. **Open reception to the complaint of a member of the Society about an improper appointment. [Correct. Members who complain do not receive open consideration, so this would challenge the information in the passage. "If any member, seeing an improper appointment in contemplation,… raise a voice against it, the ready answer is, Why should you interfere?"]**
D. The Council and the Society working in cooperation. [This is a tempting choice, but it ignores the conflict between members of the Society and the Council.]

15. The passage implies that the party is open to suggestions by the Society under which circumstances?

A. After the member of Society waits a certain length of time. [Incorrect. The Council finds a way to discredit suggestions or complaints.]
B. When the Society as a group submits a written appeal to the party. [Not supported.]
C. After the member of Society retracts his complaint. [Not supported.]
D. **None. The party stonewalls members of the Society. [Correct. "A member of Society who wishes to file a complaint to the Council is first delayed, then discounted for being out-of-date, and finally deemed a meddler."]**

16. According to the passage, when does enjoying pleasure become useful?

A. When it is sought after a day of work with no further consideration than to enjoy the pleasure itself. [Correct.]
B. When music accompanies it. [Not stated.]
C. When the object of enjoyment is imitated. [Not stated.]
D. When we feel our dispositions. [A direct quote, but not relevant.]

17. The author would most likely disagree with which of the following statements:

A. Music gives pleasure naturally. [No, he strongly agrees with this idea.]
B. Harmful pleasures are not necessarily relaxing. ["…for all those pleasures which are harmless are not only conducive to the final end of life, but serve also as relaxations;"]
C. Music is best pursued when enjoyment of it is the sole reason for hearing it. [Correct.]
D. The pleasure of an apple cannot be imitated. ["…now it happens in the other senses there is no imitation of manners; that is to say, in the touch and the taste;" Furthermore, since the question does not specify the taste or appearance of the apple, we cannot know for certain to which quality the question refers.]

18. The tone of the author is best described as:

A. high-flown. [No, not that extreme.]
B. erudite. [Correct. The author speaks in a educated tone.]
C. trite. [The author is not trite.]
D. enthusiastic. [No, the syntax and grammar are not light or enthusiastic.]

19. The passage implies that a person who lives a life of virtue and happiness must:

A. pursue pleasure, preferably in the form of music and poetry. [Not stated.]
B. live by courage and modesty, mildness and anger when appropriate. [These describe music and poetry.]
C. live by enthusiasm, courage and modesty, and seek pleasure after a day of labor. [Does not answer the question correctly.]
D. be pleasant and honorable, and enjoy what should be enjoyed, and hate what should be hated. [Correct. "It is admitted also that a happy life must be an honorable one, and a pleasant one too, since happiness consists in both these …and as virtue itself consists in rightly enjoying, loving, and hating,…"]

20. The passage suggests that the author would agree with each of the following statements EXCEPT:

A. A sculptor who molds a beautiful sculpture can experience the same pleasure as another sculptor who molds a similar sculpture. [Correct. "…thus, if any person is pleased with seeing a statue of anyone on no other account but its beauty, it is evident that the sight of the original from whence it was taken would also be pleasing…"]
B. A child's fear of a costume of a large bear is as legitimate as his fear of a real bear. [Incorrect.]
C. A sculptor and a painter looking at the same sculpture can share the same level of enjoyment. [Incorrect.]
D. A chef's enjoyment of a soup can be as pleasing as his enjoyment of a different soup. [Taste from the same object cannot be imitated, but taste from different objects could provide equal enjoyment.]

21. This passage would most likely appear in which format?

A. poetry journal. [No, too narrow.]
B. health and wellness publication. [Correct.]
C. newspaper editorial. [Too erudite to be a typical newspaper article.]
D. creative writing journal. [This is not a piece of fiction.]

22. The most likely title of this article is:

A. The Happiness of Art. (Too broad.)
B. Music and Relaxation [Correct. The overall theme is about music and relaxation.]
C. Enjoy Life the Right Way. (Too broad.)
D. Happiness and Virtue. (Too narrow.)

23. The main argument of the passage is that:

A. Stamps represent the artistic progress of the country that made it. [Not always true since the author indicates a stamp may represent the lack of artistic progress.]
B. Stamps are no longer indicative of the artistic status of the country by which they are issued. [False.]
C. **Stamps are the focus of the artistic efforts of a nation. [Correct. Stamps may represent artistic efforts, whether successful or not.]**
D. Stamps depict aspects of achievement for a given nation. [Too broad. The author focuses on artistic depictions.]

24. The author is most concerned about which of the following driving forces for the production of stamps?

A. strong pride of a nation. [No.]
B. **appeal to collectors. [Yes. "But too often, we fear, these picture stamps are produced merely with a view to their ready salability to collectors."]**
C. artistic expression of a society. [The author is not concerned about artistic expression.]
D. promotion of natural resources. [The author is not concerned about promotion of natural resources.]

25. The passage suggests that a stamp bearing only inscriptions might be considered each of the following EXCEPT:

A. unpopular with collectors, probably because of their inability to read them. [This is possible.]
B. **valuable, because stamps of this nature are rare. [Correct. The author does not mention that stamps with inscriptions alone are rare.]**
C. interesting for their crude and curious designs. [This is possible.]
D. informative, because they may reveal which cultures coexist. [This is possible.]

26. The author would expect the designs of stamps to suggest many things, EXCEPT the:

A. power of nations. ["Egypt has her sphinx and pyramids…"]
B. technology of civilizations. ["The stamps of Rhodesia and the Congo Free State depict the advance of civilization."]
C. **prosperous future of a society. [Yes. No example pointed to the future of a country.]**
D. scenic grandeur of a country. ["Sometimes this is due to national pride and occasionally it is intended to draw attention to the resources and natural wonders of a country."]

27. Which of the following examples would best describe a contemporary stamp?

A. A stamp made in Brazil depicting life on the Amazon River. [No. There needs to be a difference between the place depicted, and the place of production.]
B. A late issue of the Eiffel Tower made in Paris. [No. There needs to be a difference between the place depicted, and the place of production.]
C. **A late issue from the Tonga islands but made in London. [Correct. "More frequently than not, these brilliant labels are the product of a distant country and are no longer indicative of the artistic status of the country by which they are issued."]**
D. A stamp depicting a coat of arms with the portrait of a king. [No. There needs to be a difference between the place depicted, and the place of production.]

28. The discussion of General Lew Wallace's Fair God suggests that as men love to trace their descent back to some past greatness:

A. civilizations seek to associate a divine animal with their prosperity. [The imagery in the first paragraph depicts the founding of a nation, not its prosperity.]
B. nations take pride in their foundation at the hands of a religious leader. [Incorrect.]
C. civilizations trace their descent back to a symbol of divinity. [We cannot say for sure that the eagle is a symbol of divinity.]
D. **nations delight to associate the gods with their origin. [Correct. The imagery brings together a god with the foundation of a nation.]**

29. According to the passage, which of the following describes complete soil cultivation?

A. Barnyard liquid manure with crop-rotation, tillage and drainage. [Yes. Each element is necessary for sustainable farming as described in the passage, and barnyard liquid manure contains healthy amounts of vegetable matter.]
B. Kainite, dried blood and byproducts, bone treated with sulphuric acid, and lime with shallow tillage, drainage and crop rotation.[Shallow tillage is unhealthy for crops.]
C. Florida rocks treated with sulphuric acid, cotton-seed meal, and wood ashes with deep tillage and crop-rotation. [No. Drainage is not included in this list.]
D. Soda from Chile, muriate of potash, and lime with tillage, crop-rotation and drainage. [This excludes a source of phosphoric acid.]

30. The author would most likely agree with which of the following statements?

A. Excellent nitrogen sources are found in Germany. [No. Potash is found in Germany.]
B. The decay of organic matter is not beneficial for the soil. [No. Lime is added to the soil in order to accelerate this process.]
C. Corn and cotton use up soil nutrients faster than many other crops. [Yes. "You remember that the virgin soils contained a great deal of vegetable matter and plant food, but by the continuous growing of crops like wheat, corn, and cotton, and by constant shallow tillage, both humus and plant food have been used up."]
D. The smell of ammonia in the table is unnatural. [No. The decomposition of liquid manure into ammonia is a natural process.]

31. As implied by the passage, how would a farmer improve the quality of soil year after year?

A. Apply good tillage and crop-rotation, drain well, and add humus and plant food. [Yes. All steps will ensure fertile soil.]
B. Grow wheat in virgin soil with tillage and drainage. [No. Virgin soil will lose nutrients without replenishment.]
C. Use lime and nitrogen with crop-rotation, deep tillage, and dried blood. [This excludes drainage, potash, and phosphoric acid.]
D. Use shallow tillage in times of excess rain, along with phosphoric acid, nitrogen, and potash. [Shallow tillage allows for loss of nutrients.]

32. Which method of fertilizing would most likely incur the *greatest* cost?

A. Adding phosphoric acid from South Carolina rocks. [We cannot say for sure. The correct answer must be defendable from information in the passage.]
B. Plow under cowpeas. [The author gave no information about the cost of plowing under cowpeas.]
C. **Applying barnyard fertilizer. [Yes. The author states that raising livestock is mandatory. "There are three ways of adding humus and plant food to this lifeless land: the first way is to apply barnyard manure (to adopt this method means that livestock raising must be a part of all farming)"]**
D. Adding cotton-seed meal. [The author gave no information about the cost of adding cotton-seed meal.]

33. During the rainy season, a prudent farmer would take which action?

A. Apply lime and extra kainite. [No. Loss of nitrogen must be prevented.]
B. **Apply ammonium sulphate in small quantities at various intervals. [Yes. "Nitrate of soda is soluble in water and may therefore be washed away before being used by plants. For this reason it should be applied in small quantities and at intervals of a few weeks."]**
C. Apply extra nitrogen in each application in the form of cotton-seed meal. [No. Nitrogen should be applied in small quantities.]
D. Apply less drainage so as to minimize nutrients washing away. [No. The passage never suggests that drainage should be diminished. In fact, less drainage may lead to flooding.]

34. Given that a plot of land contains dead soil, how would the author propose to revive it?

A. Remove the bad soil, add solid barnyard manure mixed with lime, then apply drainage and crop-rotation with tillage. [No. This is missing nitrogen which is contained mostly in the liquid portion.]
B. **Remove the bad soil, add fresh soil mixed with liquid manure, then apply drainage and crop-rotation with tillage. [Yes. This contains all the nutrients and methods for sustainable crops.]**
C. Remove the bad soil, add humus and plant food, then apply crop-rotation with tillage. [No. Drainage is absent from this list.]
D. Remove the bad soil, add ammonium sulphate and kainite, then apply drainage and crop-rotation with tillage. [No. Phosphoric acid is absent from this list.]

Answers and Explanations

35. According to the passage, the author would most likely agree with which statement?

A. Chiefs of nations contributed to the design of their heraldic arms. [This was not indicated in the passage.]
B. Heraldic arms were the exclusive domain of knights, chiefs, and sovereigns. [No. "Honorable ordinaries were the original marks of distinction bestowed by sovereigns on subjects that had become eminent for their services, either in the council or the field of battle."]
C. Honorable marks of distinction were bestowed primarily for achievements in battle. [Incorrect. Honorable marks were bestowed also for excellent council. "Honorable ordinaries were the original marks of distinction bestowed by sovereigns on subjects that had become eminent for their services, either in the council or the field of battle."]
D. **Heraldic arms never included offensive signs. [Correct. "Sovereigns and Lords of Europe should be distinguished, all of whom were ardent in maintaining the honor of the several nations to which they belonged, was a matter of great nicety, and it was properly entrusted to the Heralds who invented signs of honor which could not be construed into offense…"]**

36. A sovereign would feel disinclined to bestow the figure of a lion on a person who performed which action?

A. Remaining on the battlefield after the battle has ended. ["Was it a warrior, who, though victorious, was still engaged in struggling with the foes of his sovereign, the lion rampant was considered a proper emblem of the hero."]
B. **Punishing enemies after they have surrendered. [Correct. Showing clemency was valued in heraldry. "Armorists have introduced lions to denote the attributes of majesty, might, and clemency, subduing those that resist, and sparing those that yield to authority."]**
C. Jailing instigators of an uprising. [This is an example of "subduing those that resist."]
D. Parading through a conquered town. [This could fall under the category of majesty, and is not the best answer.]

37. Which of the following attributes did not contribute directly to the origination and evolution of heraldry?

A. **pomp [Correct. Pomp was never mentioned in the passage.]**
B. military fame [This was indicated in the passage.]
C. loyalty to sovereigns [This was indicated in the passage.]
D. extraordinary council [This was indicated in the passage.]

38. Suppose that the King of Spain conquered the Kingdom of Prussia. Which of the following repercussions would most likely occur?

A. The Prussian Arms of Dominion would change. [Incorrect, because Arms of Dominion do not change by a change of control. "…and could not properly be altered by a change of dynasty."]
B. Cities of Prussia would change their Arms of Community. [Incorrect.]
C. The King of Spain would grant the Arms of Concession to the King of Prussia. [Incorrect.]
D. **The Spanish Arms of Pretension would change. [The kingdom of Spain adds new territory under its dominion. "Arms of Pretension were those of kingdoms, provinces, or territories to which a prince or lord had some claim, and which he added to his own, though the kingdoms or territories were governed by a foreign king or lord…"]**

39. According to the passage, which of the following depict historic uses of emblazoned arms?
   I.   Mark of distinction.
   II.   Device of organization.
   III. Sign of submission.

A. I only. [Yes, but II is also correct.]
B. III only. [This is never indicated.]
C. **I and II only. [Mark of distinction and device of organization are correct: "When numerous armies engaged in the expeditions to the Holy Land, consisting of the troops of twenty different nations, they were obliged to adopt some ensign or mark in order to marshal the vassals under the banners of the various leaders." "The regulation of the symbols whereby the Sovereigns and Lords of Europe should be distinguished…"]**
D. I, II, and III. [Statement III is not correct.]

40. Which modern-day practice most nearly captures the purpose and significance of heraldic arms of the past?

A. **Emblems representing military squadrons. [This is the best answer because heraldic arms were used extensively in battle to organize armies. "When numerous armies engaged in the expeditions to the Holy Land, consisting of the troops of twenty different nations, they were obliged to adopt some ensign or mark in order to marshal the vassals under the banners of the various leaders… The passion for military fame which prevailed at this period…"]**
B. Coat of arms representing family names. [Heraldic arms were used for reasons beyond mere family identifiers.]
C. Seals representing presidents of nations. [This is a good answer as heraldic arms represented "chiefs of different nations," but is not the best answer.]
D. Symbols representing historic events found on currency. [This is not very relevant.]

VERBAL TEST 7

ANSWERS AND EXPLANATIONS

1. Suppose that the nobility enjoyed exemption from taxation. Which of the following statements, if true, would best represent a justification of this exemption by Turgot?

   A. **Nobles are bound to yield military service without pay. [Correct. Turgot believes in the principle of equality and balanced contribution. "The expenses of government having for their object the interests of all, all should contribute to them; and the more advantages a man has, the more that man should contribute."]**
   B. Nobles are privileged and not bound to any service. [Incorrect. Turgot believes in the principle of equality and balanced contribution. Everyone should contribute to society in one way or another.]
   C. Taxation without representation is unjust. [No.]
   D. Nobles comprise the government, and a government cannot tax itself. [Not supported.]

2. The passage indicates that the Parliament of Paris believed:

   A. equality of duties among citizens preserves civil society. [Incorrect.]
   B. an imbalance between rich and poor exists in every society. [This is a vague statement.]
   C. **positions of privilege is a birthright. [Correct. The passage indicates birthright is an important consideration. "The first rule of justice is to preserve to every one what belongs to him: this rule consists, not only in preserving the rights of property, but still more in preserving those belonging to the person, which arise from the prerogative of birth and of position…"]**
   D. the caste system establishes a foundation for society. [This may be suggested, but choice C is the best answer.]

3. The author suggests that commoners in France challenged feudalism when they:

   A. obtained wealth from economic reform. [This is not suggested.]
   B. gained control of provinces and towns. [While this might make sense, the author does not offer this as the main reason.]
   C. gained access to the judiciary, and discovered that the nobility could not harm them. [A tempting choice, but the author implies that the nobility possessed weapons. Thus, the nobility was in a position to harm commoners whether or not commoners were armed or not.]
   D. **gained access to weaponry, and discovered that the Church could neither harm nor aid them. [Correct. Commoners were held back by fear of clergy, and by a lack of weapons. "The essence of feudalism was a gradation of rank, in the nature of caste, based upon fear. The clergy were privileged because the laity believed that they could work miracles, and could dispense something more vital even than life and death. The nobility were privileged because they were resistless in war. Therefore, the nobility could impose all sorts of burdens upon those who were unarmed."]**

4. The tone of the author can be best described as:

A. neutral. [Yes. The author does not express opinions in this passage.]
B. insightful. [The author does not make any interesting deductions.]
C. critical. [The author is not critical.]
D. cynical. [The author is not cynical.]

5. Positions of privilege are described as "titles... bought for money." Turgot does not support this practice most likely because it:

A. challenges the principle of order. [A tempting choice, but Turgot disagrees with inequality, not disorder.]
B. supports the Parliament of Paris. [Incorrect.]
C. broadens the gap between rich and poor. [This answer has the right idea, but choice D is the better choice. Always pick the most clear and direct answer.]
D. transforms the judiciary into a caste. [Correct. The author in paragraph 1 reveals the unjust nature of the judiciary, and then follows with the example of Turgot in paragraph 2 as a proponent of the "principle of equality."]

6. The author suggests that the study of matter:

A. conceals itself in the mind. [Truth conceals itself in the mind, not the study of matter.]
B. eludes the philosophers of his day. [Incorrect.]
C. is similar to the study of Beauty. [Incorrect.]
D. leads to endless experiments. [Correct. Matter has infinite divisions and thus can undergo infinite philosophical tests and experiments. "…in short, to pursue matter through its infinite divisions, and wander in its dark labyrinths, is the employment of the philosophy in vogue."]

7. Which of the following would suggest that the author's concern about the pursuit of Truth is exaggerated?

A. A physicist offers theories on light behavior. [Not the best answer.]
B. A linguist proposes a new philosophy on truth. [Correct. The author states that the study of words obscures truth. So a linguist who succeeds at defining truth would suggest the author's concern does not apply universally. "But, though the mischief arising from the study of words is prodigious, we must not consider it as the only cause of darkening the splendors of Truth, and obstructing the free diffusion of her light."]
C. A psychologist reveals the subconscious meanings of joy. [Incorrect.]
D. A philosopher creates a new philosophy. [Not the best answer.]

8. Which of the following statements is inconsistent with information in the passage?

A. Language, when used improperly, alters the nature of truth. [Correct. The passage states that truth can never be altered. "For, since all truth is eternal, its nature can never be altered by transposition…"]
B. Matter influences how we discover Beauty. [This is consistent. "But here it is requisite to observe that our ascent to this region of Beauty must be made by gradual advances, for, from our association with matter, it is impossible to pass directly…"]
C. A genius does not bother with the study of details. [This is consistent. "To a genius, indeed, truly modern, with whom the crucible and the air-pump are alone the standards of Truth, such an attempt must appear ridiculous in the extreme…"]
D. The study of details can waste intellectual energy. [This is supported. "…and the science of universals, permanent and fixed, must be superior to the knowledge of particulars, fleeting and frail…"]

9. The assertion that the "science of universals, permanent and fixed, must be superior to the knowledge of particulars," is:

A. supported by Plotinus. [We do not know whether Plotinus supported this view.]
B. **supported by the author's discussion of the perception of Beauty. [The author states that the study of Beauty is like that of matter. "But here it is requisite to observe that our ascent to this region of Beauty must be made by gradual advances, for, from our association with matter, it is impossible to pass directly, and without a medium, to such transcendent perfection…"]**
C. contradicted by the author's own use of language. [No.]
D. contradicted by examples set by the Heroes of Philosophy. [The Heroes of Philosophy studied Truth, and is not relevant here.]

10. Suppose the author uses the metaphor "like the brightness which is seen on the summit of mountains previous to the rising of the sun." This image describes most likely the concept of:

A. Truth, and the process of discovering it. [Incorrect.]
B. Language, and the process of understanding it. [Incorrect.]
C. **Beauty, and the process of perceiving it. [Correct. The perception of beauty has a strong corporeal aspect. "…the perception of the beautiful… even while connected with a corporeal nature."]**
D. Intellect, and the process of using it. [Incorrect.]

11. The reference to "the gaudy colors of butterflies" suggests that the author:

A. dislikes frail things. [This is an exaggeration. The author never expresses personal distaste in the passage.]
B. disapproves of nature's wisdom. [The author never suggests this.]
C. **does not want to spend time defining minutia. [Correct. The author finds particulars to be fleeting and frail. "…the science of universals, permanent and fixed, must be superior to the knowledge of particulars, fleeting and frail…"]**
D. has another definition of Beauty. [Possibly, but choice C is much more clear and direct.]

12. This passage was written most likely for:

A. biologists. [This is not a piece on biology. It is philosophical.]
B. philosophers. [A tempting choice, but the author does emphasize those who "study" which suggests that, perhaps, the target reader is a student of philosophy.]
C. **students. [The passage makes a few references to those who study. "…every lover of truth will only study a language for the purpose of procuring the wisdom it contains… and he who wishes to emulate their glory and participate in their wisdom, will study their doctrines more than their language… But, though the mischief arising from the study of words is prodigious…"]**
D. psychologists. [This is not a piece on psychology. It is philosophical.]

Answers and Explanations

13. According to the passage, each geological feature can serve as a site for a mineral vein EXCEPT:

A. porous and soluble rock. [Incorrect. "Thus in soluble rocks, such as limestones, joints enlarged by percolating water are sometimes filled with metalliferous deposits…"]
B. fissure veins. [Incorrect. "While fissure veins are the most important of mineral veins…"]
C. sandstone. [Incorrect. "Even a porous aquifer may be made the seat of mineral deposits, as in the case of some copper-bearing and silver-bearing sandstones of New Mexico."]
D. **gold ores. [Correct. Gold is not a porous or water-soluble mineral, and thus cannot serve as a site for mineral vein formation.]**

14. In the context of the passage, the word lithologically most nearly refers to

A. **composition and texture. [Correct. Following the word lithological, the author discusses various kinds of rock which suggests their different compositions and textures.]**
B. elevation. [No. There is no suggestion of elevation.]
C. geographical location. [No. It is obvious that the author is referring to different geographical locations and would not have to state this.]
D. fossil content. [Incorrect. The author states that these locations contain similar fossils. "All would be similar, however, in the fossils which they contain."]

15. The author suggests which of the following about geology?

A. **The zone of cementation exists below the zone of solution. [Correct. "As the surface of the land is slowly lowered by weathering and running water, the zone of solution is lowered at an equal rate and encroaches constantly on the zone of cementation."]**
B. Two categories of veins exist. [No. Fissure veins are a type of mineral vein. "While fissure veins are the most important of mineral veins…"]
C. Fossils of fish bones prove that the strata were laid after the appearance of mammals. [This is not a correct answer because the author states this directly, and is thus not considered a suggestion. "The presence of the bones of whales and other marine mammals would prove that the strata were laid after the appearance of mammals upon earth…"]
D. Zinc deposits would most likely appear in the zone of cementation. [Incorrect. The author does not provide enough information to make this suggestion.]

16. The author provides an explanation or example in the passage for each of the following EXCEPT:

A. Lower levels of veins may contain large amounts of silver. [While the author never mentions silver, he does explain how lower levels of veins accumulate minerals (ie. silver). "The minerals of veins are therefore constantly being dissolved along their upper portions and carried down the fissures by ground water to lower levels, where they are redeposited."]

B. The origin of igneous rock and lava. [The author does explain this. "Earth movements fracturing deeply the rocks of the crust, the intrusion of heated masses, the circulation of underground waters…"]

C. The absolute age of strata can be determined. [Correct. The author only offers a way to determine one age relative to another, but not absolute age. "The presence of the bones of whales and other marine mammals would prove that the strata were laid after the appearance of mammals upon earth, and imbedded relics of man would give a still closer approximation to their age. In the same way we correlate the earlier geological formations."]

D. The formation of fissure veins. [The author does explain this. "The minerals of veins are therefore constantly being dissolved along their upper portions and carried down the fissures by ground water to lower levels, where they are redeposited."]

17. The author would agree with which of the following statements:

A. Gold from igneous rock is useless. [Correct. "…gold and other metals from igneous rock, but in this widely diffused condition they are wholly useless to man."]

B. Mineral veins are the original source of the metals of veins. [Incorrect. Igneous rock is the original source. "It is to the igneous rocks that we may look for the original source of the metals of veins."]

C. Western Europe and Georgia share similar rock formations. [Incorrect. They share similar fossils. "The correlation of formations by means of fossils may be explained by the formations now being deposited about the north Atlantic. Lithologically they are extremely various."]

D. New Mexico and the Mississippi valley share similar metal deposits. [Incorrect. "…the lead and zinc deposits of the upper Mississippi valley. Even a porous aquifer may be made the seat of mineral deposits, as in the case of some copper-bearing and silver-bearing sandstones of New Mexico."]

18. According to the passage, which of the following fossil findings would the author consider most unexpected?

A. Two different plant specimens in the same strata of earth from the same geographic region. [Incorrect. The author would expect to find many different plants within the same region in any given era.]

B. Two different plant specimens in two different strata of earth from different geographic regions. [Incorrect. The author would expect to find many different plants within various regions of different eras.]

C. Two similar plant specimens in two different strata of earth from the same geographic region. [Correct. Finding two similar fossils in the same region in the same rock strata is expected. But finding two similar fossils in the same region of different eras would be unexpected. Plants and animals are expected to change with time. "Making all due allowance for differences in species due to local differences in climate and other physical causes, it would still be plain that plants and animals so similar lived at the same period of time, and that the formations in which their remains were imbedded were contemporaneous in a broad way."]

D. Two similar plant specimens in two similar strata of earth from different geographic regions. [Not the correct answer. The author might expect to find similar plants from two different locations as long as they came from the same era.]

19. The main argument of the passage is that:

A. resentment goes further than vague verbal outbursts of temper. [This may be true, but does not capture the full argument of the passage.]
B. the natural and instinctive desire of the human animal is to find a scapegoat. [This captures the main argument of the author.]
C. whatever sort of misfortune falls upon people, they will always blame something. [A tempting choice, but the author emphasizes that the desire to find a scapegoat is instinctual.]
D. we have ourselves to blame for misfortune. [This is also a tempting choice, but ignores the inborn nature to find a scapegoat.]

20. According to the passage, the response of the crowd towards Cinna the poet:

A. Helps confirm that our ancestors believed there was always someone to blame. [May be true, but is not the main message from this example.]
B. Reveals the true unreasonable nature of people. [A poor choice.]
C. Embodies the universal impulse of humanity. [Correct. The main idea of the author is that the habit of finding a scapegoat is universal.]
D. Supports the claim that resentment prefers to blame an innocent victim. [May be true, but is not the main message from this example.]

21. Which of the following scenarios would the author find most surprising?

A. A teenage girl stomping the sidewalk where she tripped. [Incorrect. The author would not be surprised by her reaction.]
B. A cab driver blaming his flat tire on the black bird that flew across his window. [Incorrect. The author would not be surprised by his reaction.]
C. A boy suspecting that his dead relative turned out the lights during a thunder storm. [Incorrect. The author would not be surprised by his reaction.]
D. A professor arguing with his wife, and kicking his dog for trying to follow him out of the house. [Correct. The author trusts that the most educated in society will not give in to the temptation of finding a scapegoat. "…and though we ourselves have mostly got beyond that stage, yet the habit it engendered in our race remains ingrained in the nervous system, so that none but a few of the naturally highest and most civilized dispositions have really outgrown it"]

22. Which of the following statements, if true, would most *strengthen* the author's argument about scapegoats:

A. **The Athenians kept a small collection of public scapegoats always in stock, waiting to be sacrificed at a moment's notice. [Correct. "The fact is, the death is regarded as a misfortune, and somebody must be blamed for it. Heaven has provided scapegoats."]**
B. The Romans persecuted scapegoats without a fair trial. [No.]
C. The Byzantines forbade scapegoats from entering politics. [Not relevant.]
D. The Saracens punished public officers who habitually blamed others. [This would weaken the author's argument.]

23. According to one chief of a village, "all deaths that occur in life are violent deaths, and are brought about by human or superhuman agency." Upon finding his brother dead on the ground, this chief would probably:

A. call for a physician to diagnose the probable cause of death. [No. The author believes that "none but a few of the naturally highest and most civilized dispositions have really outgrown it"]
B. call for an officer to hunt down the person responsible. [The author believes that the person who feels violated will seek revenge directly.]
C. **put in jail the person at the crime scene. [Yes. This is an example of taking direct action against the perceived perpetrator.]**
D. assign a witch-finder to disclose the evil spirit at work. [No. The person who feels cheated takes direct action.]

24. The overall theme of the passage is that:

A. Economic stability is the groundwork for social protection. [This ignores the focus on insurance.]
B. Of the many forms of financial relation among men, none is more important than insurance. [The author does not hold this extreme opinion.]
C. **The protection and social cooperation of insurance depends on economic stability. [Yes. Insurance and social cooperation are the focus of the passage, and both depend on stability.]**
D. Eternal vigilance prevents war and calamity. [The author never claims that eternal vigilance will go so far as to prevent war.]

25. Which of the following statements, if true, could explain excessive insurance claims in times of war in a given country?

A. A large proportion of artisans and upper class did not participate in war. [If they did not participate in war and suffer losses, then they would have no reason to file claims.]
B. Group policies began to subject members to physical examinations. [This is misleading and irrelevant.]
C. **A large proportion of students and well-paid men were first to enlist. [Correct. The most likely men with insurance would suffer losses by enlisting first in war. "In its direct relation, war destroys those who to the underwriter represent the "best risks," the men most valuable to themselves and thus most valuable to the community."]**
D. A large proportion of uninsured men died in the war. [If they were uninsured, they would not file claims.]

26. Which factors threaten the business of insurance?
   I.   increase of loans.
   II. exhaustion of reserves.
   III. the precarious nature of investment.

A. I only. [Statements I, II, and II are correct.]
B. II only. [No.]
C. I and III only. [No.]
D. **I, II, and III. [Insurance companies must have reserve funds, so if these were depleted this would threaten the business of insurance. An increase of loans would place more burden on insurance companies. Investment is a difficult enterprise to predict. "Enforced loans from the reserve fund of insurance companies to the state mean the depreciation of reserves... War conditions mean insecurity of investment."]**

27. The author probably views life insurance as:

A. essentially altruistic. [Correct. "In every regard, the business of insurance is naturally allied with the forces that make for peace... The same remark applies in some degree to every honorable or constructive business."]
B. a necessary yet risky utility. [The author does not indicate insurance is necessary.]
C. a selfish service. [Incorrect. The author views insurance as beneficial.]
D. surreptitious. [Incorrect. The author views insurance as beneficial.]

28. According to the passage, which of the following statements can be inferred about fire insurance?

A. All fire insurance contracts in foreign nations are held in abeyance until the close of war. [Correct. "Such funds are probably never actually confiscated but held in abeyance until the close of the war. This is another form of the ever present "military necessity," which seizes men's property with little more compunction than it shows in seizing men's bodies."]
B. Based on a sliding scale, lower and upper class pay the same fire insurance premiums. [The "sliding scale" was mentioned in the passage, but this statement is not justified by the information provided.]
C. Fire insurance policies are scaled down automatically in the event of a fire. [We cannot know for sure.]
D. Fire insurance policies are not as prone to the effects of war as those of life insurance. [No. This is not supported by the passage.]

29. Which of the following statements about business during times of war reinforces the views of the author?

A. Many businesses feel unsafe about investing in bonds. [Correct. "War conditions mean insecurity of investment. In war, all bonds are liable to become scraps of paper..."]
B. Businesses scale down during times of war. [This is not discussed in the passage.]
C. Insurance companies create an economic environment that does not foster peace. [False. The opposite is true. "In every regard, the business of insurance is naturally allied with the forces that make for peace..."]
D. War slowly destroys business and economic welfare. [Not necessarily.]

30. The passage suggests that the people who stand guard at all times for the security of business should be like:

A. firemen extinguishing a fire. [Incorrect. The author states that these people should not be like firemen.]
B. fireproof building material. [Correct. The author says that such men should prevent trouble before problems occur. "Such men should stand guard against the influences that work toward conflict. Those who work for peace should be not "firemen to be called in to put out the fire" already started through the negligence of business men..."]
C. policemen investigating crimes. [Incorrect.]
D. a magnifying glass. [No, this was not suggested.]

Answers and Explanations

31. Which of the following describes the logical organization of the passage?

A. A main idea is presented, followed by several examples that support that idea. [Incorrect. A main argument is never stated by the author.]

B. Four main examples are presented, followed by the main argument. [Incorrect. A main argument is never stated by the author.]

C. Four main examples are presented with major arguments weaved into them. [Incorrect. Main arguments are never provided by the author.]

D. Four different examples are introduced to form an overall impression. [Correct. The author never presents an overall argument. Instead, the author provides details about various examples to give an overall impression of colonial life.]

32. According to the passage, grains seeded in each of the following would most likely result in an indifferent crop EXCEPT:

A. spacious soil. [Correct. "These plants required space in which to develop their full growth. A tobacco plant could be set or a hill of corn planted wherever a little loose dirt could be found."]

B. land prepared by Indians. [No. "Some English grains were seeded in the cleared land near Hampton and Newport News but these old fields, abandoned by the Indians, were also near to exhaustion. An 'indifferent crop' was reported."]

C. newly cleared forest. [Incorrect. "Newly cleared forests left the soil full of stumps and roots."]

D. any cleared land. [No. As indicated above, certain kinds of cleared land were poor in quality. "Some English grains were seeded in the cleared land near Hampton and Newport News but these old fields, abandoned by the Indians, were also near to exhaustion. An 'indifferent crop' was reported."]

33. Suppose the government fixed the price of sweet potatoes at one hundred and fifty pounds sterling per one thousand pounds. Such a decision would most likely indicate:

A. Adequate land was cleared for farming potatoes. [Incorrect. The adequate clearing of land does not guarantee favorable growing conditions. Choice D is the better choice.]

B. A drop in price of commodities competing with sweet potatoes. [No. This might make intuitive sense, but is not discussed.]

C. A rise in the number of sweet potato producers. [No. This might make intuitive sense, but is not discussed.]

D. Very dependable growing conditions. [Correct. Prices become fixed when the quality of the commodity becomes highly dependable, which arises from dependable growing conditions. "…in 1661, provision was made for importing some flax seed from England. No price was fixed, in 1666, on 'flax by reason of the uncertainty of the quality.'"]

34. Each of the following statements would conflict with the author's understanding of commodities in Colonial America, EXCEPT:

A. Historians understood the utility of all livestock. [This conflicts with the author's understanding of commodities in Colonial America. "Hogs contributed more to the material welfare of the Jamestown Colony than historians have generally recognized."]
B. Food given to livestock was suitable for colonists. [This conflicts with the author's understanding of commodities in Colonial America. "The roots of tuckahoe, often as large as a man's arm, contain a crystalline acid that burns the mouth of a human being like fire. After a few trials, hogs seem to relish it."]
C. **Colonists struggled to grow oats. [Correct. The colonists struggled to grow grains. "As already noted, the initial attempts of the colonists to grow the grains with which they had been accustomed in England came to naught. They were familiar with wheat, rye, barley and oats."]**
D. Colonists elected to grow hemp and flax. [This conflicts with the author's understanding of commodities in Colonial America. "It was also ordered that every tithable person should produce one pound of dressed hemp and one pound of dressed flax or two pounds of either annually."]

35. Suppose the colonists brought donkeys from England to Jamestown instead of horses. The most likely reaction the colonists would have to this animal would be:

A. Acceptance, because they would cost less than horses. [No. This might make sense, but the passage gives us no information regarding the price of donkeys.]
B. Relief, because donkeys could pull the wooden plows. [Incorrect. Wooden plows were fragile and were ineffective against stumps, despite how they were pulled.]
C. **Disappointment, because there were few burdens to carry. [Correct. The passage states clearly that there were few burdens to carry. Thus, any beast of burden could not serve much utility. "They were of little use as beasts of burden as there were few burdens to carry."]**
D. Frustration, because donkeys would die before reaching the mountains. [No. This might make sense, but the passage gives us no information regarding the stamina of donkeys.]

36. The priests who follow the Zend-Avesta best illustrate the author's point that:

A. Religion cannot teach the philosophical or grammatical aspects of language. [Not true.]
B. Superstition allows one to have influence over others. [This does not best answer the question.]
C. Learning religion with knowledge of philosophy and grammar is respectable. [No. The author never suggests this.]
D. **Language is not a prerequisite for knowledge. [Correct. "There are, perhaps, a dozen among the whole body of professional priests who lay claim to a knowledge of the Zend-Avesta: but the only respect in which they are superior to their brethren is, that they have learnt the meanings of the words of the books as they are taught, without knowing the language, either philosophically or grammatically."]**

37. Which of the following statements, if true, would most *strengthen* the argument of The Liberals?

A. Passages from the Zend-Avesta have been found in recent versions of the Zurthosht. [No. The correct answer must show authority in the original books.]
B. The Parsis of India have come to agreement on the authority of the Zend-Avesta. [Agreement would not prove original authority of the Zurthosht, which The Reformers question.]
C. **The practice of rubbing Nirang on one's body has been found in the original books of Zurthosht. [Yes. If true, this would attack the argument of The Reformers that there is no authority in the original books.]**
D. The Reformers retract their accusations of bigotry and weakness. [Retreat does not strengthen an argument.]

38. The Oxford English Dictionary defines religion as "a pursuit or interest followed with devotion." If the author were to include this description in the passage, it would probably be used to:

A. illustrate the point that followers of a religion remain faithful despite eventual misunderstandings and corruption. [No. This is an exaggeration.]
B. emphasize that the integrity and lessons of a religion dwindle over time. [No. This is an exaggeration.]
C. explain the author's admiration for the Zoroaster religion. [No. The quote would not suggest admiration.]
D. **support the point that followers of Zoroaster remain loyal to their faith. [Yes. "...with an unhesitating fervor such as is seldom to be found in larger religious communities."]**

39. The reference to Nirang shows primarily that:

A. There is disagreement among priests about Zoroastrian practices. [Correct. The author uses the Nirang example to focus on a major point of contention.]

B. Priests who follow the Zend-Avesta are superstitious. [No. The author does not suggest superstition.]

C. The author favors the views of The Reformers. [The author does not take a clear side.]

D. There is no authority whatever in the original books of Zurthosht. [This is never indicated.]

40. According to the passage, The Reformers would disagree with each of the following ideas EXCEPT:

A. Unclean practices do not belong in their religion. [The Reformers would probably disagree with this claim.]

B. The books of Zurthosht are not the highest authority in matters of faith, law, and morality. [The Reformers would probably disagree with this claim.]

C. Knowing the philosophy of a culture is important to knowing its religion. [The Reformers would probably disagree with this claim.]

D. The Liberals have made progress, but are small-minded. [The Reformers agree with this claim. "The Reformers have found themselves strengthened by the intolerant bigotry and the weakness of the arguments of their opponents."]

LIST OF ANSWERS

QUICK REFERENCE

Test 1

Passage I
1. C
2. D
3. C
4. A
5. A

Passage II
6. C
7. D
8. B
9. C
10. A
11. A

Passage III
12. A
13. A
14. C
15. B
16. C
17. B
18. D

Passage IV
19. C
20. D
21. A
22. C
23. A
24. C

Passage V
25. C
26. A
27. D
28. B
29. C

Passage VI
30. D
31. D
32. A
33. B
34. C

Passage VII
35. B
36. A
37. C
38. D
39. A
40. C

———

Test 2

Passage I
1. A
2. D
3. B
4. D
5. A

Passage II
6. D
7. A
8. B
9. D
10. B
11. C

Passage III
12. C
13. B
14. D
15. C
16. C

Passage IV
17. B
18. C
19. D
20. A
21. C

Passage V
22. D
23. B
24. A
25. A
26. D
27. B
28. B

Passage VI
29. B
30. B
31. C
32. A
33. D
34. C

Passage VII
35. B
36. B
37. D
38. C
39. C
40. C

———

Test 3

Passage I
1. C
2. B
3. A
4. D
5. D
6. D

Passage II
7. B
8. D
9. A
10. D
11. A
12. B

Passage III
13. A
14. C
15. B
16. A
17. A
18. C

Passage IV
19. A
20. B
21. C
22. B
23. A
24. C

Passage V
25. C
26. B
27. D
28. D
29. A

Passage VI
30. C
31. D
32. C
33. C
34. A
35. D

Passage VII
36. C
37. D
38. A
39. C
40. A

———

Test 4

Passage I
1. A
2. D
3. B
4. C
5. D
6. B

Passage II
7. A
8. C
9. D
10. C
11. A
12. B
13. A

Passage III
14. D
15. C
16. D
17. C
18. B
19. B

Passage IV
20. D
21. B
22. B
23. C
24. C

Passage V
25. D
26. C
27. B
28. C
29. A
30. A

Passage VI
31. B
32. C
33. A
34. C
35. C

Passage VII
36. A
37. B
38. D
39. C
40. B

———

List of Answers: Quick Reference

Test 5

Passage I
1. B
2. C
3. C
4. A
5. A

Passage II
6. A
7. D
8. B
9. D
10. A
11. C

Passage III
12. A
13. C
14. D
15. D
16. A

Passage IV
17. C
18. A
19. A
20. D
21. C
22. D
23. B

Passage V
24. D
25. D
26. C
27. D
28. A

Passage VI
29. B
30. D
31. C
32. D
33. A
34. A

Passage VII
35. D
36. D
37. A
38. B
39. A
40. C

Test 6

Passage I
1. D
2. A
3. B
4. B
5. D

Passage II
6. D
7. A
8. A
9. B
10. C

Passage III
11. B
12. B
13. D
14. C
15. D

Passage IV
16. A
17. C
18. B
19. D
20. A
21. B
22. B

Passage V
23. C
24. B
25. B
26. C
27. C
28. D

Passage VI
29. A
30. C
31. A
32. C
33. B
34. B

Passage VII
35. D
36. B
37. A
38. D
39. C
40. A

Test 7

Passage I
1. A
2. C
3. D
4. A
5. D

Passage II
6. D
7. B
8. A
9. B
10. C
11. C
12. C

Passage III
13. D
14. A
15. A
16. C
17. A
18. C

Passage IV
19. B
20. C
21. D
22. A
23. C

Passage V
24. C
25. C
26. D
27. A
28. A
29. A
30. B

Passage VI
31. D
32. A
33. D
34. C
35. C

Passage VII
36. D
37. C
38. D
39. A
40. A